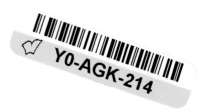

WINDOW OF OPPORTUNITY

Living with the Reality of Parkinson's and the Threat of Dementia

KIRK W. HALL

PYGMY BOOKS

Smaller. Smarter.

A Division of North Slope Publications

PYGMY BOOKS
Smaller. Smarter.
A Division of North Slope Publications

Window of Opportunity: Living with the Reality of Parkinson's and the Threat of Dementia
Copyright © 2013 Kirk W. Hall
ISBN 978-0-9842063-4-6

Other books by Kirk Hall
Carson and His Shaky Paws Grampa (Innovo Publishing, 2011)
Carina and Her Care Partner Gramma (Innovo Publishing, 2013)

For more information or to order, visit http://www.innovopublishing.com/Featured-Book-Shaky-Paws-Grampa.html

Published by Pygmy Books; a division of North Slope Publications
Woodland Park, CO

Page layout design by Marcie Miller Art

Dedication

To my wife, Linda, with all my love
and
To all my brothers and sisters in the Parkinson's community

CONTENTS

FOREWORD

The first time I met Kirk Hall was in November of 2008. In retrospect, I think it is fair to say that this meeting shaped both of our lives in ways that neither of us would have predicted at the time. I think it is also fair to say that it began a relationship that has moved far beyond what I learned about in medical school classes on communication as the "doctor-patient relationship."

I was just four months into my grown-up job as an assistant professor of neurology at the University of Colorado following more than ten years of school, residency, and fellowships. Despite all this preparatory work, I was still very much in the midst of figuring out what I was doing with my career. Still, I was not totally without direction. Having done fellowships in behavioral neurology (the neurology of problems with thinking, memory, and behavior, particularly dementia) and movement disorders (the neurology of problems with motor control, including tremor and Parkinson's disease), I was committed to doing work at the crossroads of these two fields. Being done with training meant that it was now up to me to determine what that further work would look like. I had just started doing research on non-motor symptoms in Parkinson's disease. Although this may sound focused, *non-motor symptoms* refers to any and all symptoms other than shaking, slowness, and stiffness (e.g., thinking and memory problems, hallucinations, depression, anxiety, constipation, pain, fatigue, insomnia, etc.).

Kirk was also at a crossroads in his life. He too was at the beginning of a journey that would involve the meeting of behavioral neurology and movement disorders. And despite the fact that he did not choose the medical conditions that led to our meeting, he too was faced with the dilemma of how he was going to live his life with them. Kirk was referred to me by the movement disorder neurologists who were taking care of his tremor to deal with his non-motor symptoms, which at that time included changes in thinking and memory, fatigue, and depression. Although I'm sure my notes from that visit contained a wealth of medical information, including his physical examination and neuropsychological test results, I don't think those notes (or most medical records, for that matter) captured what was really important in our interaction as people.

To begin with, the notes imply that I (the physician) am the expert and Kirk (the patient) is the beneficiary and subject of my knowledge. I think one of the many values of this book is that it turns this common wisdom on its head. Kirk *lives with* the symptoms I read and write about. He is an expert on this subject because he *is* the subject.

I remember that Kirk was anxious, and that his anxiety was centered around the changes he noticed in his thinking and memory. Scared may be an even better word for what he felt, as it implies a normal reaction to something scary rather than an abnormal reaction to something that should be easy to accept. For many people, the prospect of losing one's memory, of someday not recognizing your spouse and children, is more frightening even than death. Kirk was not afraid to be vulnerable and share his fears with me then, and he was equally candid when I invited him to speak as part of a patient roundtable discussion in front of 60 doctors and other health care providers. This vulnerability has been one of his many gifts to me and the Parkinson's community, a gift that was a driving force for this book: to take those parts of Parkinson's that are scariest and talk about them openly.

I remember reassuring him at that time that he did not have dementia and that I expected he would have many good years ahead of him. I think it was during this discussion that he first brought up the idea of writing a few books and that I first encouraged him to do so. I could tell him he had a window of opportunity that he could choose to use, but neither of us could know how long it would last. Kirk didn't just take the opportunity, he ran with it. Since that meeting he has led two Parkinson's support groups; written three books; and become an advocate for Parkinson's research, a blogger, an advocate for patients, and a national speaker. This book is important not just for the messages it contains, but as a message itself: an inspiring example of opportunities seized from a place where many would have given up hope.

Kirk is a deeply spiritual man who values his faith and draws upon it as a source of strength and inspiration. To talk about such things in our secular age seems taboo, particularly in a book on a medical topic. But despite the increasing use of technology in medicine, doctors ultimately take care of people, not diseases. When dealing with serious, progressive, and life-altering illnesses, caring means asking people about their hopes and fears, understanding their beliefs, and helping them reconnect with their sources of strength and meaning. This type of work is not currently well supported in our medical system, as it (of course) takes time, has no insurance billing category, and is not for the weak of heart.

Since my first meeting with Kirk, I have gone on to obtain grant funding to better understand the causes of dementia in Parkinson's disease, with the goal of developing improved treatments, and have started one of the first team-based palliative care clinics for Parkinson's disease in the United States. Kirk has become a local and national leader as a patient advocate. I am proud to write the foreword to this book and hope that Kirk inspires you as much as he has me.

—Benzi Kluger, MD, MS

Associate Professor of Neurology and Psychiatry

Director, Movement Disorders Center

University of Colorado, Denver

August 2013

ACKNOWLEDGMENTS

I had the benefit of help and support in the writing of this book, which was originally conceived in 2009 and completed, after struggling through 40-plus drafts, in late 2013. In its earliest stages, I received advice and encouragement from Leon Wirth, Jane Terry, and Susan Mathis, all of whom were employed by or consultants at Focus on the Family at that time. I think it was 2010 when I first mentioned the idea to Dr. Kluger, who offered to be my "medical consultant." I can recall bouncing ideas off Joel Havemann (author of *A Life Shaken,* Johns Hopkins, 2002), who is a good example of the friends I have made as a result of my interest in writing.

Special thanks go to Gerry Benedict for his generous assistance that enabled me to overcome the frustration of early "false summits." I am also indebted to Kate Kelsall, Leon Wirth,

Becky White, Jon Stamford, Angela Taylor, Barbara Snelgrove, and Linda Szabo and Janis Jarvis (my sisters), as well as my wife, Linda, for their review and helpful suggestions regarding this manuscript. There are many people I should thank for their support during the time I was writing this book (though some didn't know about it), including John Corcoran, Cheryl Siefert, Valerie Graham, Donna Miller, Karlin Schroeder, Madhavi Rao, Patti Meese, Margaret Anne Coles, Terry Bailey, and my sons, Kevin and Brian Hall. I would not have been able to complete this book without the dedication and expertise of my independent editor, Brooke Graves, who has come to know me so well that she is able to discern what I want to say when I am unable to say it myself.

Words cannot express my gratitude to Dr. Benzi Kluger, for his patience, expertise, encouragement, thoughtful counsel, and sensitivity to my concerns and needs; as well as to my wife, Linda, for being my partner on this journey, recognizing how much this project meant to me, and "giving me space" to complete it.

Finally, I need to acknowledge that none of this, for whatever it is worth, would have been possible without the grace of God.

INTRODUCTION

I was diagnosed with Parkinson's disease (PD) in 2008 at the age of 59. I am now 65 years old. A neurological exam in 2012 confirmed that I had also developed amnestic mild cognitive impairment (aMCI),[1] a condition characterized by memory (amnestic) problems more severe than normal based on age and education but not serious enough to affect daily life. This condition often precedes Alzheimer's disease,[2] Lewy body dementia,[3] or Parkinson's disease dementia.[4] Clearly not good news, but not really a shock either, due to cognitive symptoms I had experienced since shortly after my PD diagnosis.

I first had the idea to write this book during the summer of 2009 and have been wrestling with it, to one degree or another, ever since. I'm not sure why I thought this was a good idea. One of the reasons may have been that it was important to me because of my fears about my own future. Since then I have had the opportunity to meet many people with Parkinson's (PWPs) and have consistently found that, for many of them, fear of developing dementia was their primary concern.

Most people know very little about PD unless they have had family or friends with the disease. Even then, their knowledge is generally limited to the impact of PD on motor functions, such as trembling or slowed movement (*bradykinesia*). Few know about the non-motor symptoms related to PD or are aware that, for many PWPs, these are often more troubling than motor symptoms. High on the list is the slowed thinking (*bradyphrenia*) that comes with the PD package for most, if not all, PWPs. Few subjects strike fear into our hearts like the fear of cognitive decline. Will it progress to dementia? If so, what does that look like? Are we talking about Alzheimer's or something else? Might I end up unable to communicate with or even recognize those I love most? What is the prognosis for this condition?

Until recently, cognition problems associated with PD had been discussed mostly in whispers and behind closed doors by both the medical community and PWPs. Even now, this subject is only beginning to get the attention it deserves. It remains a topic that many doctors are reluctant to discuss, making it difficult for

PWPs, care partners, and families to get direct answers to their questions.

During the summer of 2008, I mentioned my concerns about the cognitive problems I had been experiencing to a "veteran" PWP (she had nine years under her belt at that point). She suggested that I read a book titled *Life in the Balance*[5] about Dr. Thomas Graboys, a highly regarded and successful cardiologist in Boston, and his experience with both PD and Lewy body dementia.

I was struck by the unflinching honesty and courage that it took for Dr. Graboys (with the help of Peter Zheutlin) to write his book. In describing the context for how he became aware of having these diseases, he freely admits that he wishes he had communicated differently with loved ones and associates. He talks about how these diseases, in different ways, affected his relationships at many levels, including those he had with patients. He mourns the opportunity missed by many colleagues in this age of industrialized medicine to develop personal relationships with patients that provide comfort to patients as well as a very useful context for providing a superior level of care. He includes heart-wrenching notes from family members who share the very real emotional impact on their lives made by the changes they saw in Tom. In the chapter titled "End Game," Tom speaks to the undesirable options he may be faced with (including assisted suicide) and his own internal debate about the right course of action for all concerned. I admire that, even after all he has been through, Tom chose a message of hope, courage, and perseverance, as well as the importance of finding a purpose, for the final chapter of his book.

Though we have never met and my only interactions with him have been a few short emails, I consider Tom to be a friend— perhaps because we have shared similar illness experiences and seem to agree on a wide range of subjects, but even more because of the ways in which he has provided me with encouragement and support. In April 2009, I sent him an email thanking him for writing his book and shared how much it had helped me. I also told him about a writing project I was working on at the time (a personal memoir). He has given me permission to share his incredibly inspirational and motivating return email, which provides a window into the impact of his dementia:

From: Graboys, Thomas Barr, M.D.

Sent: Monday, April 06, 2009 11:02 AM

To: Kirk Hall

Subject: RE: thank you

Bravo tto you mr hall and congrates on comoleting 8 chapters..writing as your can onlyimprove your situation.. it will be a legacy to your famiry.keepit up so important to keep your mind and body stimultated...keep it up!

My bestTom

Thomas B. Graboys, MD

Professor of Medicine

Harvard Medical School

Tom also mentioned in that final chapter that he was very encouraged by improvement in cognitive function and mood he experienced after taking Namenda (memantine)[6] (a drug prescribed for moderate to severe dementias). When my wife and I visited the National Institutes of Health's National Institute of Neurological Disorders and Stroke (NIH/NINDS) during October 2012 for me to participate in PD clinical research, they conducted a full review of my condition. With regard to my aMCI, the doctors recommended Namenda in conjunction with the Exelon patch[7] (which I had started using in September 2011). At my next appointment with my movement disorder neurologist at the University of Colorado Hospital in March 2013, Dr. Benzi

Kluger recommended that I add Namenda to my regimen; he said that some patients were finding the use of Namenda in conjunction with the Exelon patch to be helpful. I remembered what NINDS had told me and the positive comments from Dr. Graboys and agreed to give it a try.

I have been taking Namenda since April 2013 and have experienced noticeable improvements in clarity, acuity, mood, and working memory.[8] I had been getting discouraged about whether I was ever going to be able to write a book that would meet my expectations, but now am reasonably confident that Namenda has provided me with a "window of opportunity" to complete this task that has come to mean so much to me. Eventually I realized that this was just another example of God's presence in my life.

This book focuses on my personal experience with PD and related cognition problems, but it includes information and ideas that I hope will be interesting or useful to PWPs and their families. While it is not my primary objective, I hope it will also provide useful insights to the medical and research community.

At some point on this journey, I began to realize that what I was experiencing was *not* all bad news, and I want to emphasize this. My fears about the future were knocked off center stage by the opportunities I was being given to meet and develop relationships with other PWPs and care partners as well as other people in the PD world, including individuals employed by PD organizations, doctors, and research scientists. Thankfully, I realized that I was being given an opportunity to at least try to have a positive impact on others in my position. This, in conjunction with my faith and the love of my family and friends, has made a world of difference in my outlook. I truly feel extraordinarily blessed.

Chapter 1: Crossroads

My wife, Linda, and I decided to take a camping trip during the weekend of August 17, 2007, to celebrate our 38th wedding anniversary, which was coming up on August 23. We had become fairly avid tent campers and hikers in our 13 years of living in Colorado and had visited quite a few different places. For this occasion, we chose a campground at the base of Mt. Elbert, the highest "fourteener" (a mountain of 14,000 feet or more in elevation) in Colorado. After a first night in a somewhat mediocre campsite, we moved to an idyllic one that must have been about an acre in size, with many lodgepole pines, by a stream that rushed down from the mountain. We took some short hikes on Saturday with our sheltie, Little Fox, and enjoyed relaxing with the symphony of the cascading water as a backdrop. We decided we would get up early the next day and hike up at least part of the mountain.

The sunrise was spectacular on Sunday morning, and the north Mt. Elbert trailhead beckoned only a few hundred yards away. We grabbed our hiking poles, water, and backpacks and got started. Although our campground was at 10,000 feet, the summit was at 14,443 feet, so we had no real intention of "summitting." We left Little Fox at our campsite because we were concerned about how he might handle the altitude. It took us a couple hours to make our way up the steep trail through the forest to the timberline at about 11,000 feet. The trail looked foreboding ahead as it wound through steep, rocky terrain. We were already breathing hard after short distances and considered turning back. However, we met some people already on their way down who encouraged us, telling us the climb was well worth the effort. We decided to go on a bit further.

Breathing became increasingly difficult as we continued our climb. We developed a strategy of picking a destination at progressively shorter distances ahead as our goal where we stopped to recover. We probably would have turned around and headed back down if not for the intermittent passers-by who told us how glad we would be when we got to the top. At some point, we threw caution to the wind and decided to go for it.

The trail got increasingly steep and treacherous (we later learned that there was a southern route that was far less challenging) and we were disappointed by a couple "false summits" where we reached a crest only to find that we still had quite a distance left to climb. At that point, though, we had determined to meet the challenge and persevered until we reached the top at about noon. We put on the jackets we had packed in our backpacks, drank our water, and ate our lunch as snow flew lightly around us and we enjoyed the view with a handful of other hearty souls. We had someone take a picture of us to commemorate the moment. We both felt exhausted, but also exhilarated by the sense of unexpected accomplishment.

While at the summit, we learned of the southern route and decided to take it in spite of the fact that we would have to hike miles across the base of the mountain when we got down. The weather looked good and we still seemed to have sufficient water. We were feeling good about ourselves as we started back down on a much easier trail.

The problem with going downhill is that it uses different muscles and also puts pressure on the knees and hips. Our toes started to become sore from rubbing against our boots. We became a little more concerned when dark clouds suddenly appeared on the horizon. The wind quickly increased to near-gale force as we heard the first echoes of thunder. Realizing that we were above treeline and totally exposed, we began to run. I was really starting to hurt and lagged behind Linda. We stopped to put on our rain parkas when it began to sleet heavily. We continued our soggy jog for what seemed like forever until the rain finally stopped. We were above treeline and knew that we were still in danger, but stopped to rest for a few minutes. I attempted to sit on a rock, failing to realize that the terrain was still very steep, and almost fell over backward.

An additional problem developed as we realized we were almost out of water. It was going to take another couple hours just to get to the base, then another three hours to traverse back to our campground. Two younger men whom we had seen farther up the mountain came by and asked if we were all right. We explained our water situation and asked if they knew of a place where we could get a refill. They were parked at a lot close to the base and offered to share their supply! Though we were now sore and thoroughly exhausted, we made it to the bottom and hiked the six miles back to our tent, where we found Little

Fox anxiously waiting. By then it was 7:00 p.m.—we had been gone for 13 hours.

After resting and drinking what seemed like a gallon of water each, we started to pack up so that we could begin the drive home. As we were loading the car, the men who had given us their water pulled up in their car. We had told them where we were camped and they drove well out of their way to make sure we had gotten back safely. We were so touched and grateful for such amazing kindness!

As I reflect on this experience now, I think that it was significant well beyond what I realized at the time. I had been excited about the achievement of climbing the mountain and surviving the tribulations of the trip down. I was mystified, and continue to be amazed, by the unexpected concern shown by those two strangers who we will never see again.

I now clearly recognize God's hand in these events. We had a chance to prove to ourselves that we can accomplish more than we may have thought possible if we persevere. We saw that when the going gets tough and our plans prove inadequate, there is still hope. And, even when hope begins to dwindle, God will provide. As events continue to unfold, this knowledge is a source of great comfort and encouragement to Linda and me.

Within months after climbing that peak, Linda and I would enter a valley unlike any we had encountered before. In that valley we would find an unexpected crossroads. We would have no map to help us decide which way to go or forecast what we would find at the end of our journey. This would not be the last time we would forge ahead armed only with our trust in God.

Chapter 2: Life before Parkinson's

I was born November 12, 1948, in Cleveland, Ohio, to parents who were about 27 years old and already had a 2-year old daughter. (Another sister followed two years later.) My dad had been a staff sergeant in the Army Air Corps, who was stationed in Egypt and Italy during World War II and then attended Ohio State courtesy of the GI Bill. Most of my relatives lived in the Cleveland area, and both grandfathers worked for the New York Central railroad. My heritage is 50% German and 50% UK (English, Irish, Scottish, and Welsh).

We had a nomadic lifestyle in the early years, living in seven different locations in northern Ohio before moving into a rural home on subdivided farmland between Akron and Canton in 1956. The farmer whose land we had bought delivered eggs to us and gave me the opportunity to help him and his son with combining and hay baling. During those years, my sisters, friends, and I spent a fair amount of time building forts, playing sports, and hanging out in barns and corncribs.

I was generally healthy growing up. In fact, I received a special award as a senior in high school for perfect attendance since sixth grade. I did have the normal assortment of childhood illnesses, plus a bout of scarlet fever when I was four or five. During childhood, I got lots of exercise through sports and play, and I continued to be active as an adult with running, tennis, skiing, biking, golf, swimming, weight training, hiking, yardwork, and more. However, I have taken blood pressure medication since I was about 30 years old and have been evaluated periodically by cardiologists since my early thirties, due to my dad's problems with heart attacks and stroke when he was in his fifties (he was overweight and smoked three packs a day). Also, while growing up, I was exposed to fertilizers and pesticides, due to the farm and rural environment as well as the fact that my dad was an avid gardener. I also drank well water during these years (exposure to pesticides and drinking well water have both been identified as risk factors for the development of PD).

Religion was not a big deal in my immediate family, though it clearly was to my grandparents. We did attend church and Sunday school sporadically and I joined a high school Bible study group for a time during my junior year. I remained ambivalent about faith until a life-changing event led me to become a believer and be baptized when I was about 30. This event occurred during a time when I was having a variety of personal problems involving flawed choices. Linda and I talked about it, and she asked me, in so many words, what I used as my "compass" for making these choices/decisions. She reminded me that she relied on her faith for direction. In typical Linda fashion, she planted a seed (as she would many times in the future) that germinated in my mind. One Sunday, after she had left for the church she was attending with our boys, I spontaneously decided to go to a church I had seen in the area, but never attended. I drove to this church not knowing what time services were held, and arrived as the pastor was beginning his sermon. His topic that day was about the problems people face when they "build their house on sand instead of rock" (Matthew 7:24-27). I was totally blown away. Since then I have been actively involved in churches in the communities where we have lived, including parish councils, youth group activities, and choir. Many of our closest friends are people we have met through the churches we have attended. As time has gone by, I have learned to depend on

God and have been consistently amazed by His impact on our lives.

My dad's career was mainly in wholesale sales management and department store merchandising and management. We moved back to the Cleveland area for my senior year in high school due to one of his job changes. My passions growing up were sports (Little League baseball, basketball, and golf teams in high school and college) and music. Personal highlights included pitching a no-hitter and all-star game in Little League, being captain of my high school golf team, being chosen for the All-County Select Choir my junior year, and playing the lead in my senior class play.

After graduation, I attended Ohio State University. There I met Linda during the first quarter of our first year; we were married in 1969, before our senior year. After a brief stint in the Army, when I trained as an infantry officer at Ft. Benning, Georgia, we lived a nomadic lifestyle much as my family had done. However, since we both preferred to avoid winter (she grew up in Buffalo), we started in Tampa before moving to Sarasota/Gainesville, Florida (where our first son was born in 1972), and Charlotte, North Carolina. I was in retail variety store management during those years—a tough life at best—

and decided to make a change and move into the consumer electronics industry, where I spent the next 20 years, off and on (I spent 1980-1981 obtaining an MBA), in different positions. During those years we lived in Grand Rapids and Detroit, Michigan (where our second son was born in 1975), and Buffalo, New York (where I went to graduate school), before relocating to Oakland, New Jersey, after graduation. While living in New Jersey from 1982-1994, the most interesting and productive phase of my career was spent in Manhattan working for the corporate merchandising offices of Federated Department Stores (where I was ultimately responsible for the collective consumer electronics businesses of chains that included Burdine's, Rich's, Lazarus, Foley's, and Bloomingdale's) and as a vice president in the direct mail catalog division (the fifth largest direct mail catalog business at that time) of American Express.

While I was at American Express, I experienced a number of notable neurological developments. In 1991, I was at an executive strategic planning training session in Princeton when I noticed that my hand was shaking as I carried a plate of food. My doctor told me it was essential tremor (ET), which I apparently inherited from my mom, and it was much more noticeable in my left hand. He assured me that it was not Parkinson's, based on my symptoms and absence of a family history of PD, but just to be sure, I made an appointment with a neurologist, who concurred with my first doctor. The tremor was mild at that time, but became more troublesome as the years went by, especially when I was eating, drinking, or trying to putt. In the mid-2000s, I also noticed weakness in my neck that caused head tremor—another ET symptom.

I worked in American Express's World Financial Center headquarters in Manhattan, which was directly across the street from the World Trade Center building that was bombed on February 26, 1993. This was a traumatic event for all of us who were there at that time. I can still vividly recall sitting in a meeting in the middle of the building on the 42nd floor at Amex and feeling the shock wave before hearing the enormous blast. All of us in that room spent anxious moments wondering where this explosion had taken place and wondering if our building was about to collapse. As we all know now, the blast caused great damage and actually came close to accomplishing the goal of bringing down WTC1. Needless to say, when I witnessed the devastation that took place on September 11, 2001, while watching *Good Morning America* as I got ready to go to work, I was horrified beyond words like everyone else. However, it somehow affected me more deeply and personally, probably because I worked in such close proximity to the WTC for almost six years. For the first few of those years, I often took the Path train from Hoboken into WTC1. I was in both towers frequently for lunch or to take visitors sightseeing. I had been to the top and felt the fear I always feel when looking down from great heights. I had also felt the fear of a possible imminent collapse of the Amex building in 1993 when the first WTC blast occurred, which probably gave me a hint of what it must have been like for those souls who perished on 9/11. I had put it off, but in 2012 I finally visited Ground Zero where rebuilding was under way. I suppose it was at least somewhat cathartic for me to visit this place, have my memories, shed my tears, and say my prayers. However, I know in my heart that I will never be the same.

It may also be noteworthy that the first WTC bombing was one in a series of significant and stressful life events starting in 1992. I lost my dad to pancreatic cancer in August 1992 and a young man who worked for me to AIDS the following year. My business had become increasingly challenging and stressful, primarily due to changes taking place within Amex. I was under pressure due to budget constraints, layoffs, and increased responsibilities. Then, there was a car accident in April 1993.

While at the furniture market in High Point (one of the businesses for which I was then responsible), my boss was driving back to the hotel after dinner one evening when we were hit head-on by a drunk driver at an intersection in Greensboro, North Carolina. I am embarrassed to admit that I was not wearing a seat belt (I recall having my suit coat on and being concerned about getting it wrinkled); had it not been for my long legs wedged under the dash, I would likely have gone through the windshield. As it was, my head hit the windshield with enough force to crack it (the windshield, not my head—guess my wife was right about me being hard-headed); my suit coat, while unwrinkled, got covered with blood. We were released after being checked out at the local emergency room, but I recall feeling like someone had grabbed me by the ankles and slammed me against a wall a few times. More important than that, I saw it as a wakeup call.

Also in 1992, I started to experience what I came to describe as "brown-outs" (like what happens in New York City during a heat wave in the summer, when the lights dim because of a power drop-off due to high use of air conditioning). I would be sitting in a meeting, in the middle of talking, when it seemed like the world around me slowed down briefly and I would have trouble getting the words out of my mouth—kind of like living in slow motion. I don't know if this was noticeable to others (no one ever mentioned it), but it certainly was to me. This happened on more than a few occasions over a period of about a year, I think. Toward the end of 1992 and continuing into 1993, I also experienced problems with swallowing and had to take an inordinate amount of time while eating and use extra caution taking pills. Interestingly, both problems disappeared after I left Amex in 1994. However, the swallowing difficulties resurfaced while I was staying in a hotel on Times Square for business purposes in 1998. It took about two months for the problem to subside, during which time I ate a lot of bananas and drank a lot of protein shakes (good way to lose weight, but not fun). I talked to my doctor about this problem and ended up at the local hospital where my swallowing apparatus was thoroughly checked and pronounced to be in good working order. The cause of my problem was never determined.

After my car-accident "wakeup call" in April 1993, I told God that He now had my undivided attention and I was ready to rearrange my priorities. After considering a variety of possibilities, my wife and I decided to make quality of life our priority for the first time. We felt that we had lots of options regarding where we could live, as long as I was close enough to civilization to be able to use my experience to make a living (I was 45 at the time and nowhere near being able to retire). Both boys were in college at the University of Colorado, so we were free to make a move. I was able to negotiate terms that allowed me to manage a mutually acceptable transition out of Amex, and we made the move to Colorado, a place the whole family had come to love during family ski vacations, in early 1994.

As it turned out, I was probably too cavalier about my career when we chose to move to Colorado, but in looking back, I wouldn't change our decision. The boys both ended up staying here (in the Denver area) and getting married and we now have six beautiful grandchildren. We were able to buy the house of our dreams that was a perfect fit with our Colorado lifestyle: a beautiful log "cabin" surrounded by huge Ponderosa pines. We built a huge redwood deck on the back overlooking Pikes Peak and the Air Force Academy (a view we also enjoyed inside through the many windows in our great room). Inside, we renovated the kitchen, great room, and bathrooms, giving them a rustic feel to match the rest of the house. We have enjoyed many wonderful tent camping and hiking trips in the mountains, not to mention lots of world-class skiing in jaw-droppingly beautiful locations. We were able to join a private golf club as well as a tennis club that enabled my wife to continue her outstanding competitive exploits. I was able to expand my singing involvement to include performances with the Colorado Springs Symphony, as well as solo work at both sons' weddings, church services, funerals, weddings, and our local music association's Christmas concerts.

Starting in 1999, I became one of two managing partners for a small career transition services company in Colorado Springs. This type of small business was uncharted territory for me, but after a couple of years of struggling to execute the "vision," we were making excellent progress and expanded our operation to include Denver and the entire Front Range. We were in the midst of planning for further expansion in the Rocky Mountain region when the economy went seriously sour in mid-2003.

My inexperience in the entrepreneurial arena (and bad luck) led to me personally losing a good deal of money, and the business was sold to an investor. Worst of all, I ended up in a four-year legal battle with my ex-partner over his liberal use of company funds to pay his own bills toward the end of our partnership (only the tip of the iceberg, as it turned out). I was disappointed to learn that I was not as good a judge of character and trustworthiness as I had thought. I was determined that he should be held accountable for his actions and was able to develop a strong case with the help of our company accountant and my attorney. However, once again I received a "reality check" lesson when the DA elected not to bring my case to trial. What was a huge deal for me was obviously not a big enough fish for him to want to fry. I ended up having to settle for an insignificant amount so that I could pay my legal bills and put this affair behind me.

Clearly, the stress from this legal business affected me, as did earlier events at American Express. However, there is no way to know if any particular event triggered the PD. Following my initial ET diagnosis, I was evaluated for different reasons over the years, and was never told that I even "might" have PD. But I now know that PD is a tough thing to diagnose, especially in the early stages. With the benefit of hindsight, I can now see that there were signs along the way, in addition to the essential tremor. For example, I started to notice changes in my senses of smell and taste in late 2003. On a number of occasions, when I was under stress, my whole body would shake in a way that was unlike anything I had experienced before. I had to work harder to stay organized and found it harder to think clearly under pressure. In 2007, as our 38th wedding anniversary approached and we planned the Mt. Elbert hike described in chapter 1, I lost my publishing marketing director position without cause due to a management change and budget cuts. I was struggling and my faith was being tested.

It is interesting for me to look back on these events and try to make sense of them. My early years of exposure to toxins and well water in rural Ohio could be significant. There is a generally consistent higher rate of occurrence of PD in rural states. From a pollution standpoint, I lived in metropolitan/industrial areas including Cleveland, Akron (the air used to stink around Akron from the rubber factories), Detroit, and NYC. I started consuming alcoholic beverages in college; although I only infrequently drank significant amounts, I nevertheless added a source of body toxicity by doing so. I was undoubtedly eating foods that had been sprayed or processed with toxic substances as well.

Clearly, "neurological events" were occurring in the early 1990s, including my ET diagnosis, the "brown-outs," and the swallowing issues. Although I wrote those off as caused by stress at the time, especially given the fact that all but the ET subsided after I left Amex (with only the swallowing problem reoccurring under the stress of going back to NYC), my sense now is that there was an underlying predisposition to Parkinson's that only surfaced under significant duress. It is also possible that trauma incurred from the blow to my head during the car accident in 1993, and another during a snow skiing accident in 2004, could be a factor, but there is no evidence to support such a speculation. I do think that my lifetime exposure to toxins had a cumulative effect on my brain and nervous system as well. The changes in smell and taste in 2003 were a clear "red flag" based on what I know now.

Stress almost certainly has played a role. Without going into detail, at least some of my teen years were abnormally stressful, as were the early 1990s and most of the period from 2003-2008. Of course, stress is relative: What is stressful to one person may not be (or may be less so) to another person. Given this, it may be significant that I am and have always had a sensitive nature. Life in the corporate world could well have taken a different toll on me than it would have on someone with a "thicker skin." Of course, all of this is at least somewhat speculative, but my guess is that if we were playing "Battleship," I would have at least hit, if not sunk, a few boats.

Chapter 3: The Elephant in the Room

Nine months after our Mt. Elbert mountain climbing experience, in May 2008, I was in a business meeting in Colorado Springs. At that time, I was marketing director for an agency that provided marketing and advertising consulting for organizations throughout the United States. This meeting was not all that different from hundreds I had attended (or led) in my 38-year career. However, the circumstances were different in that I had been diagnosed with Parkinson's disease (PD) about a month earlier. I had made an appointment during April 2008 with a movement disorder neurologist[9] (MDN) at the University of Colorado Hospital (UCH) for an evaluation of my essential tremor[10] condition (a troublesome condition involving potentially debilitating "action tremor"), which was the only thing to which I could attribute the intense fatigue and disproportionate reaction to stress I had been experiencing. Much to my surprise, I was told that I now was dealing with early-stage PD in addition to ET.

During the course of that May meeting, I started having trouble "processing" the things I was hearing and became literally unable to participate. At that time, I did not really know what to expect with regard to PD symptoms, other than having been told that "everyone is different" in terms of their symptoms. Like most others, I spent only a few minutes with my doctor following my initial diagnosis and was basically on my own until my next appointment in three months. I decided that I would learn as much as I could about PD, through books, other PWPs, support groups, doctors, and the Internet, hoping that this would help me to better understand the changes I was experiencing. In the coming weeks and months I would learn a great deal that was enlightening and helpful, but found very little information pertaining to cognitive issues.

The problems with processing and storage of verbal information continued. It seemed that I would do OK for a while and then gradually just "shut down." This would have been distressing in any case, but was even harder to accept based on the experience I had in managing high levels of responsibility where meetings were a way of life.

One day I was working at my desk and answering the phone while others were at lunch, working on my computer and taking a variety of messages at the same time. I must have reached an "overload" point when I looked for a message I had written for one of my co-workers so that I could leave it in his office for him. I checked all over my desk, on the floor, in the wastebasket and couldn't find it anywhere. Finally, I decided to check in his office, though I had no recollection of taking it there (around the corner and down the hall). I opened his door and there it was on his desk.

I had an interview with another company during this time. It was a company I had been interested in for several years, so part of me was looking forward to it. However, I didn't feel particularly comfortable about going to the interview due to the problems I had been having. Plus, I knew that the stress of a new job (if I got an offer) was not going to be a good thing. I rehearsed for the interview quite a bit because I didn't trust my memory. Unfortunately, another strange "memory event" occurred while I was driving to the interview. I knew that a turn I had to make was coming up. I couldn't remember anything else until I became aware that I didn't know where I was. I had no recollection of passing the point where I was supposed to turn. I kept going straight and eventually made it to the right place, but was a little bit late (not my style). I went through the interview process, but did not do well and did not get an offer. In hindsight, that was for the best.

The theme of "sensory overload"[11] keeps coming up in my attempts to describe the nature of my problems. During a vacation in California with my wife, one of my sons, and his four children, we spent a day at Disneyland. I was still having a good time during the "Jungle Cruise" (one of my favorites at Disney World, which we had been to twice many years ago). However, toward the end I started to sense that same "overloaded" feeling, and I began to process more slowly until I literally became totally dependent on Linda to lead me from one venue to the next. I guess I should not have been surprised that this happened, given the crowds of people, high volume of ambient noise, and so much other concentrated sensory bombardment.

On a variety of occasions going back to the first year I was diagnosed, my doctors described me as a "high-functioning" patient. (I suspect that this may be their code word for "pain in the neck" because of all the questions I asked.) Still, I have been told that intelligence and level of education are thought to play a role in delaying progression of cognitive/memory problems connected with PD.[12] This subject was addressed at the World Parkinson Congress[13] in Montreal during October 2013 by Dr. Janis Miyasaki, who stated that, while typical patients tend to deteriorate at a fairly steady rate over time in terms of their ability to function at previous levels, high-functioning patients tend to deteriorate much more slowly over time and then decline more precipitously.

Obviously, the potential for onset of PD-related dementia is my "elephant in the room." It took an epiphany of sorts to stop focusing on the possible unpleasant outcomes associated with this information. Dr. Kluger's practical suggestion was that I should "keep doing what I'm doing" and "hope for the best." It was time for me to take ownership of the situation and decide what to do next.

Chapter 4: Learning Curve

During the month after the meeting where I first became aware of my cognitive problems, I experienced dizziness, increased fatigue, mild balance issues, headaches, and mental "fogginess." My problems with retaining verbal information continued. It is anyone's guess how much of this was related to depression and/or anxiety. I know I was spending too much time worrying about the PD and its possible implications for the future. This culminated in early June with a trip to the emergency room at Penrose St. Francis Hospital when my symptoms intensified at work. They did a complete blood workup and a brain CT scan. This started a chain of various tests with specialists to find the problem or at least rule things out. At the ER, we ruled out diabetes or a brain tumor. They suggested that I visit my ENT and a neurologist to investigate further.

The next month, I met with a local neurologist who had been highly recommended by a PD support group in Colorado Springs (more on this group later). The neurologist was unable to confirm my PD diagnosis, which was not surprising based on the fact that he is a pediatric neurologist and my symptoms were very subtle. However, he was concerned enough about my description of "cognition problems" to order a memory baseline test (MBT). He also expressed concern about abnormal balance issues and ordered a new brain MRI (he felt this was a good idea because of the greater detail it would yield compared to the CT scan that had been done at the ER).

I also had an appointment with an ENT who had performed a sinus surgery on me in 2004. After an examination that showed no sinus problems, and a hearing test, he told me that although he could not be sure, he thought my problems were related to my central nervous system. He also ordered a VNG (videonystagmography) test to determine if I had any inner-ear problems. My guess is that they use this test at "Gitmo" to get prisoners to talk. They blow first cool air and then warm air into each ear for about 60 seconds each. After about 30 seconds each time, my left arm started to jolt intermittently like someone was electrocuting me. Needless to say, I was glad when that test was over. The results were negative.

The brain MRI and memory baseline test were done in early July. For the most part, the MBT (which was administered in the neurologist's office and took about two hours) was not problematic for me. However, I did experience difficulty when we did a verbal story memory test. It felt like the same thing that been happening to me at work. I would concentrate on what was said, but at some point stopped being able to keep up and process what was being said. As a result, I had a hard time providing details about the story afterward.

Linda and I met with my doctor at the University of Colorado Hospital again in mid-July. I asked Linda to come along because I thought she could help me remember the details of the discussion. About a month earlier, I had started keeping a timeline to help me keep track of events as they took place. When dealing with what I feel are important events, I pay a lot of attention to detail and tend to become analytical (to a fault). So, when we showed up for my appointment, I was armed with my timeline and a detailed list of symptoms, issues, and questions. My doctor did another brief PD exam and reconfirmed her diagnosis, emphasizing that the disease was in its early stage.

At that point I asked her opinion regarding my brain MRI, which she had not yet had a chance to review but had with her. She read the findings of the cover letter (written by a specialist) which indicated nothing particularly abnormal and in fact showed little change from my 2004 MRI. At that point, she plugged the MRI into her computer and, after a few moments, expressed concern.

She went on to observe that, although this was not one of her areas of expertise, there appeared to be more atrophy (atrophy or shrinkage in the brain is a normal part of aging) than would be expected for my age and that it was most evident in the frontal portions of the brain. She also pointed out some areas that she said were larger than normal (she mentioned the sylvian fissure in particular). Based on the MRI and the cognition problems I had described, she said she thought it would be a good idea for me to have an in-depth neuropsychological exam and offered to refer me to the National Jewish Medical Center (NJMC). We got an appointment for late October.

Other Approaches and Occurrences

I think it is important to point out that this was a very lonely time for me—and I suspect it may be for many others in the early stages of neurological disease. These problems are difficult (at best) to diagnose, and yet the problems people experience are real, if sometimes hard to describe accurately. It felt like nobody was really taking me seriously, even my wife. My doctors were not agreeing on my PD or the presence of brain atrophy. They were unable to help me understand what was happening with my cognition; in fact, they seemed reluctant to talk about it. Linda was concerned about my health, but she was also (justifiably) worried about our financial security. At that point, it became clear to me that I was going to have to be my own best advocate, at least for the time being.

In addition to all the doctors I was consulting, I had also joined a PD support group in Colorado Springs. The first meeting I attended reminded me of the famous bar scene from the first *Star Wars* movie. I know this sounds cruel, but it is not meant that way; I suppose it was unsettling to picture myself in their place at some point in the future. In any case, I felt like a fish out of water because my symptoms were so minor by comparison. One younger woman's frustrated, tearful comments resonated with me, though. She said that she had been diagnosed with early-stage PD and that she had had to quit her job because the stress made it impossible to do her work. She described being in a state of "limbo": unable to work and yet not qualified to receive

Social Security disability insurance (SSDI) because of the rigid definitions used by the government. While I know there have to be rules to keep people from taking advantage of this program, it seems to me that some people who should qualify for these benefits are denied simply because so many neurological diseases are so hard to diagnose.

Since I felt that I was reaching the end of my rope at work and was not independently wealthy, I tackled the problem on two related fronts by investigating SSDI and unemployment. I was not thrilled with the prospect of either, but I was looking for "any port in a storm." I went to the local Social Security office and quickly learned that my early-stage PD diagnosis was not going to qualify me for SSDI. However, I knew that any determination along those lines would depend on the neuropsychological exam and that it would likely be December before we had the results.

Once again, I met with the president of my company, who already knew of my PD diagnosis, and told him that I did not feel I could continue to work. We were able to reach an agreement for my position to be eliminated so that I would be able to apply for unemployment. He added that he hoped my situation would improve and that I would be able to return to work for them. I was greatly relieved, since I would be able to stop working at an increasingly debilitating job without having to worry about our financial security for at least six months.

A downside of all this is the way I entered into "retirement" in early August 2008. I doubt that my story is unusual, as baby boomers like me have been disproportionately affected by layoffs and downsizing over the past decade. What makes my story different is the need to stop working at a relatively young age due to serious illness. A few very thoughtful co-workers took me to lunch and gave me a nice card and gifts. It was not the fulfilling end to a storybook career that I would have liked, but I was grateful for the consideration of these folks and the knowledge that I would not have to continue working, at least for a while.

Soon after I stopped working, I started keeping a journal to record my thoughts and feelings about events as they unfolded. I backtracked to the beginning of the year to provide a more complete picture. As previously mentioned, I had already been keeping a timeline to help me keep track of important medical appointments, health changes, work information, and other important developments. I am sure that all this was related to my interest in writing "something" once I retired. I remember thinking that God may have provided me a "window of opportunity" and I wanted to make the most of it if that was the case. I wanted to write some sort of memoir for my boys— one that would be interesting but not tedious—and hoped that it might also be of interest to future generations. I also thought that I might eventually have something worthwhile to share with other PD patients, though at the time I put this idea on the back burner.

I had been advised to see a cardiologist to rule out any vascular issues and made an appointment with a medical group in Colorado Springs that I had used some years previously. The doctor listened to my description of my symptoms, my early PD diagnosis, and my previous ER experience and ENT/ neurology exams. He also reviewed my blood test results, which my primary care physician had ordered, and did a baseline EKG. He commented that my cognition problems were not related to any vascular issue. He ordered a carotid test, an echocardiogram (ECG) to make sure there were not blockages in my carotid arteries or heart valve problems, and a tilt-table test. My readings were stable throughout. In reviewing the test results, the doctor told me that I had no cardiovascular problems at that time, although he recommended another visit in six months.

By this time, driving had been problematic for a while. During the last month of work, I would often have trouble staying awake while driving home. As time went by, I was able to describe the way I felt as "mildly to moderately inebriated" all day every day. As a result, I became aware that I was concentrating harder than usual when driving (like when slightly under the influence). I knew then (and know now) that this was like a "cognitive DUI" and started being very careful about not exceeding the speed limit. In early September, I was parking the car at a shopping center and hit the car that was parked next to the spot I was pulling into. The odd thing was that I had no idea I was in any danger of hitting that car. I lost my concentration briefly. I did not just graze this other vehicle, but hit it directly enough to bring my car to an abrupt stop. Fortunately, no one (including me) was hurt, though I was shaken by the incident. I left a note on the windshield of the other car, but was never contacted (newer bumper technology is much improved and, in spite of the velocity of the contact, the only sign of the collision was my paint on the parked car's bumper).

I told Linda about the incident and we developed an unspoken agreement that she would drive whenever we were together. Since that time she has always managed to work it out so that I wouldn't be driving when our grandchildren are in the car. I understand—and wholeheartedly agree—that any risk when it comes to them is unacceptable. I continued to drive into Colorado Springs on occasion and even drove to the Denver airport in early January 2009, but mostly limited myself to driving locally to do errands and go to our club to exercise.

The decision about how to limit or when to stop driving is very difficult for PWPs, but extremely important. Accidents that are determined to have been caused by a person who chooses to drive with neurological illness can have severe legal and financial consequences. Also, the potential to seriously injure oneself, passengers, pedestrians, or other drivers has to be considered (Dr. Kluger has told me that medical testing is available to help PWPs and care partners with this decision for about $400 in many locations nationwide[14]).

Regarding exercise, I have learned that it is one of the best things I can do to slow down the progression of PD[15] (it also can create noticeable improvement for those in more advanced stages). While I was still working after my diagnosis, I ramped up my club visits to 4 or more per week, improved my conditioning, and reduced my weight to my lowest level in 15 years. I continued to work out three to four times a week after the

PD diagnosis. After I stopped working, I continued to exercise, but had too much time to think about things, get depressed, and eat too much. After a while, my metabolism couldn't keep up and I started to put on weight (definitely not a good thing, and I knew it). By the time the holidays were over, I was 20 pounds heavier. In early December, I had committed to myself and my family that I would get down to the target weight my doctor and I had talked about. Unforeseen events would complicate that plan, as it turns out. In any case, I attended a couple of spinning classes with Linda and was surprised that I did pretty well. The next day, however, I was extremely tired. Finding "balance" is a continuing challenge.

I had been encouraged by my doctor to pursue alternative strategies for improving my health, such as yoga[16] and acupuncture.[17] I had my first acupuncture appointment in early September with a practitioner who had an excellent reputation and good credentials. Based on her initial evaluation, she felt that, since I was in the early stages of PD, there was a good chance that her treatments would totally eliminate the disease. Although this was very encouraging, I remained somewhat dubious, based on my experience with chiropractors who want to have you coming in on a regular basis. I had a series of 10 treatments that involved me lying on a comfortable table with about 10 needles stuck in my head, arms, hands, and ankles (the positioning was changed based on the symptoms I reported and the therapist's sense of how I was doing). I did feel better after most of the appointments, though I wasn't sure whether it was due to the treatment or my sleeping (which I always did) for 20 to 30 minutes. The cost was about $60 per session and I did not continue when the 10 sessions were completed. It might have helped if I had continued, but I was not convinced and could not justify the expense (which was not covered by insurance).

Later in October I started physical therapy locally and also signed up for a "Therapeutic Yoga" class at our club. I spoke to the instructor who assured me that her classes would be appropriate for my situation. I took these classes until mid-December when they ended, and really enjoyed them. I would often work out upstairs for an hour or more and then come downstairs for the yoga class, which lasted 1.5 hours. My instructor assured me that she would be doing this class again and I told her I would like to participate.

Neuropsych and More

On October 28, 2008, Linda and I went to the National Jewish Medical Center in Denver for my neuropsychological exam. I was extremely nervous about this appointment, as it sounded like it would be a grueling experience with various tests lasting up to six hours. The exam was administered by a staff neuropsychologist and his assistant from 10:00 a.m.-2:15 p.m. The session started with an interview, first with both Linda and me and then just with me, that lasted about an hour. There was a 15-minute closing interview at the end. There was a lunch break from 11:45-12:30. Some tests were easy, some were challenging, and some were very difficult. It was obvious that I was having problems processing and retaining verbal information as well as with fine motor skills. The testing was much more extensive than I had received during the memory baseline test I had taken earlier, though some tests were similar. I was told that I would probably not have the results until after Thanksgiving, but the lead doctor assured me that he would provide detailed feedback to a new neurology doctor at University of Colorado Hospital— Dr. Benzi Kluger—to whom I had been referred due to my cognitive issues.

When Linda and I met with Dr. Kluger on November 17, he did have some preliminary feedback from the neuropsychologist that led him to believe that my problems might be related to depression and anxiety (not an unreasonable hypothesis based on the information he had at that time). Unfortunately, Dr. Kluger did not have all the information that would ultimately flow from the finished "neuropsych" evaluation, and he was not aware of the memory baseline test, brain MRI, or the comments about possible brain atrophy. He administered an abbreviated neuropsych exam of his own that showed no problems. He stated that he did not feel I had symptoms suggesting the potential for Alzheimer's or other dementia-type diseases. He did express concerns regarding possible depression, and recommended medication that my family doctor prescribed for me soon thereafter (I started taking an antidepressant called Wellbutrin). Toward the end of the appointment, it seemed that Dr. Kluger was starting to feel like there was possibly more to my situation than he had originally thought, and he assured me that he would talk about my case at their staff meeting that week and discuss next steps.

Of course, Linda latched on to Dr. Kluger's opinion regarding my not being at risk for Alzheimer's or anything like it; in fact, she sent out an email to family and friends sharing this good news. I was encouraged as well, but I knew that Dr. Kluger did not have the benefit of all the facts. I told Linda I would feel a lot better when we got the full neuropsych results, and clung to the hope that no significant problems would have been found.

Six weeks later, on New Year's Eve 2008 (no champagne was included), I received in the mail a nine-page letter from the National Jewish Medical Center documenting the results of the neuropsychological exam. The report included a diagnosis, based on my test results and my first UCH doctor's opinion regarding atrophy, of amnestic mild cognitive impairment (aMCI); it stated that my memory difficulties could represent the early stages of an underlying degenerative process associated with Parkinson's disease. This was not totally unexpected, as I had already been diagnosed with Parkinson's. However, I was jolted by the next comment, which read: "another neurodegenerative process such as Alzheimer's disease, Lewy body disease, or a frontotemporal dementia, may also be involved." With this information fresh in my mind, I did the sensible, mature thing by going to a New Year's Eve party and drinking way too many martinis.

One of my favorite TV commercials, run by Labatt's beer a few years ago, featured a bear playing chess in the park with an older gentleman. When the man declares "Checkmate!," the frustrated bear moans, "I did not see that coming!" This was how I felt when I received my PD diagnosis in 2008. The obsessive research that I did thereafter was helpful in many ways. The downside, especially with some of my cognition/memory research, was that I was armed with just enough information to jump to premature conclusions. I started to believe that I was in the early stages of Lewy body dementia, and of course generated a lot of anxiety for myself about that. This became a vicious cycle, as both anxiety and depression can create dementia-like symptoms. I also learned later that my low vitamin B12 levels could have contributed to symptoms I was experiencing. Place all this in a bowl and stir in the various, sometimes conflicting, cognitive impairment and cerebral atrophy feedback I was receiving, and you have a person on the verge of becoming a basket case.

I am glad that we went through the appropriate steps to rule out alternative explanations for my symptoms during this time, and that I took some positive, proactive steps such as the acupuncture, physical therapy, yoga, and exercise. I had started a self-education process that would ultimately pay dividends in terms of my ability to advocate on my own behalf as well as be helpful to others. I also started to think about my interest in writing and laying the groundwork that would enable this book to take shape.

I prayed a lot during that time that God would show me the path that He would have me follow. One day in August 2008, a few months (that seemed like a few years) after my diagnosis, I was writing in my journal about how I needed to spend more time doing things and praying for others instead of focusing so much on myself. As I wrote these words, my doorbell rang. It was a friend from church who had come by to drop off a "prayer shawl" for me. A group of ladies at church knitted these shawls and prayed over them that they might help bring peace and comfort to those who wore them. They had learned of my illness from our pastor, with whom I had met on several occasions to share my thoughts and concerns. I can't tell you how moved I was that they would do this for me! I decided at that moment to follow through on my idea to do more to help others, as these folks had done for me. I was sure it was, once again, something He was leading me to do. Still, as it turned out, it would take some time before I would be able to live up to that commitment.

Chapter 5: What's Up, Doc?

As 2009 began, I was filled with trepidation. I had really just started to accept the idea of life with PD, in spite of the conflicting opinions I had received, when I received the fresh dose of anxiety regarding cognition from my November neuropsych results.

During this time, in addition to the problems with processing and retention of verbal information that had been confirmed by the testing, I had some unusual memory lapses. For example, one day I was talking to a lady at my doctor's office about my older son's, athletic accomplishments in high school. For the life of me, I couldn't remember the third sport he lettered in three times (I remembered tennis and soccer). It was about a half hour later when I finally remembered it was ice hockey. On another occasion, I asked my son Kevin a question, then repeated the same question five minutes later. I was definitely feeling the effects of extreme uncertainty generated by the conflicting medical opinions and inability to understand what was happening to me.

I turned my attention to the atrophy question, which seemed to be a key factor related to the potential for progression to something really nasty. Based on the neuropsych results, I had been assigned to and met with Dr. Kluger at CU Anschutz (due to his expertise with both PD and cognition), but my next appointment was not until February 5. I needed to do *something* in the meantime (I felt that the clock was ticking toward some unknown conclusion and maybe I could come up with something that would help, or at least answer some questions). So, I spent a good deal of time doing Internet research regarding brain atrophy and the various dementias (educating myself and also further raising my anxiety level). I communicated with other medical professionals through friends and relatives and received a rather grim prognosis if, in fact, I was progressing toward dementia. The consensus was that there is really nothing that can be done at this time to reverse the course of these problems. Drugs such as Aricept, Namenda, and Exelon can be used in an attempt to reduce symptoms and slow progression, but results vary by individual and the medical community does not universally support their effectiveness. However, Dr. Kluger gave me hope when he shared with me that PD patients sometimes respond more positively to these medications and that exercise, mental stimulation, level of education, and continued social engagement may help slow progression. I have also been hearing recently about potential benefits from improved nutrition, as described in a book titled *Grain Brain*[18] by Dr. David Perlmutter.

During early January 2009, I started to notice and keep track of unusual "jolts" in my legs, torso, and other parts of my body. Sometimes this would happen at night, but it would also happen during the day. I had problems with a crawly, restless feeling in my legs when sitting or lying in bed that I learned was called restless leg syndrome (RLS). I also began noticing that I "startled" very easily; for example, when I was resting and Linda would wake me up, or if I was working on something and she would say something to me. Sometimes my reaction was so strong it felt like I was jumping out of my skin

I continued to have problems with fatigue and sleepiness, although I was sleeping 9 to 10 hours a night plus a nap during the day. I started to feel like I had "rechargeable batteries" that would no longer fully charge. I have had my CPAP (which I started using about eight years ago to avoid sleep apnea) checked periodically to make sure that it is not contributing to the problem. Periods of concentration, like working on the computer, reading, or driving (which I did infrequently), accentuated and exacerbated the fatigue problem. I began to notice that I would become quite irritable for brief periods of time (especially when tired). I also became confused much more easily when I was fatigued.

Nevertheless, I was determined to stay as active as I could by working out at our club and participating in winter sports like skiing and snowshoeing. Though my endurance wasn't great, I found that I was still able to downhill ski. I had been pleasantly surprised to notice the same thing with bike riding. I had seen Michael J. Fox ice-skate on one of his specials and heard him and Dr. Oz explain that, once in motion, he could skate very well; I guess that is right in line with my experiences with skiing and bike riding.

In early February 2009, at my second appointment with Dr. Kluger, he reviewed the brain MRI that had been the subject of the different interpretations from my Colorado Springs neurologist and UCH doctor and played a key role in the aMCI opinion in my neuropsychological report. His opinion was that the MRI was normal! Obviously, this was great news, but also confusing. Dr. Kluger informed me that he had expertise in this area and was confident that this MRI did not show anything problematic based on my age. I later discussed this with my neuropsychologist, who concurred with Dr. Kluger's opinion and advised that I trust Dr. Kluger's interpretation. In between appointments, I had forwarded copies of the MRI to my sister-in-law, who is a nurse in the University of Southern California student health department, who gave them to the USC neurology department for an evaluation. They also returned an opinion that the MRIs were normal and that they showed no reason for concern. This was a great relief, but still didn't help me understand what, in fact, was going on with me cognitively and what the future held for me in that regard. I had been told previously that my condition could get better, stay the same, or get worse over time. Based on the aMCI opinion, the "get worse" option was significant. With this change in the MRI interpretation, it was clear that my prospects had improved, but I was still very much in limbo. However, my wife and sister-in-law encouraged me to put my worries aside and move on, which I attempted to do.

At this same meeting with Dr. Kluger, he prescribed selegilene, my first PD medication. He also increased my dose of coenzyme Q10 (an antioxidant I had started taking in December that had been the subject of PD research) from 300 to 800 mg; suggested that I start taking the supplement l-carnitine, continue to take vitamin B12 (even borderline low levels of this vitamin can cause dementia-like symptoms), and continue to do aerobic cardio exercise for 30 minutes 5 days per week; and referred me to the hospital's integrative medicine department for fatigue evaluation. He gave me his email address so that we could keep in touch between appointments, which was a big deal for me (three months was a long time for me to wait when I had so many questions). We discussed the concerns my wife and I had about finances, and he recommended that we apply for Social Security disability insurance (SSDI). Dr. Kluger became a valued and much-appreciated partner with us that day. It would be wonderful if everyone in our position had someone like Dr. Kluger on their team.

I filled out a disability application around this time and filed it online. It was quite extensive and required digging up a lot of information on medical and employment history. I did my best to be thorough and answer all the questions as completely and honestly as possible. I had learned that most initial applications are rejected unless the situation is extremely obvious (like terminal cancer). In spite of this, based on my interpretation of their guidelines, I felt that my application would be approved. This was a key piece of the puzzle for us going forward in terms of financial security, as was our plan to sell our house (more on that later).

I was trying to put my concerns about cognition aside, but was having trouble doing so. In February, I mentioned to Linda that I thought "my assets up north were headed south." I just didn't know if the destination was South Carolina, South America, or the South Pole. I continued to experience periodic abnormal "events." One week, when we were playing golf with friends , I was playing a Titleist 3 golf ball and had another in my pocket. After teeing off, I checked my pocket and was surprised that there was only one Titleist 3 in my pocket. It took me a few moments to realize that the other was out in the fairway. Another day, I sent an email to my choir director giving her information on when I would be available to sing—and I was looking at the calendar as I wrote. Luckily I copied Linda, who emailed me to let me know I had given incorrect dates. A short time later I was working on my book. When I was done, I looked over what I had written and had to correct a number of goofy mistakes, including haven given 1970 as the year Brian and Sybil were married (in fact, it was 2000). I found it hard to put my fears aside with these kinds of incidents taking place.

During March I had my appointment in integrative medicine. In addition to exploring the fatigue question, we reviewed all my medications and supplements, addressed my nutrition, and discussed the possibility of counseling. Regarding fatigue, we found that my vitamin D level was lower than it should be and I got a vitamin shot (this started an ongoing battle, which continues today, to keep my "D" levels up, since this can affect both fatigue and cognition). I also had the opportunity to discuss my interest in a supplement I had learned about called acetyl l-carnitine. My online investigations had uncovered a research study that showed promising results in delaying onset of dementia with this supplement. The doctor checked her database and, when she found that this was correct, recommended that I take the dosage used in the research (2 grams per day).

I use this as an example of why I think it is important to participate in your medical care, especially in cases that involve "slippery subjects" like neurological disease. There is so much that is not understood in these cases and nobody knows what I am experiencing as well as I do. Therefore, I choose to learn all I can so that I can advocate for myself and also be in a position to provide helpful information to other PD patients, which is very meaningful to me.

There are few subjects that strike more fear into the hearts of older folks than Alzheimer's or dementia in general. Cancer is certainly right up there, but even that does not have the ramification of causing you to lose your ability to think, reason, remember, or recognize people you love. I am no exception. I have always considered my mind to be my best asset (which is not the same as maximizing its potential, but that's another story). Maybe that's why the medical community has only recently begun to be forthright in its discussion of this subject as relates to PD. When I first started experiencing these problems, I was able to learn facts about the various dementias, but very little about what I could expect as a PD patient. Since then, it seems that the field has had an epiphany of sorts and that non-motor symptoms, including cognition and memory, are being recognized as at least equally problematic for many PD patients—if not more so. This doesn't remove all fear from these subjects, but I would rather be armed with the facts than stick my head in the sand and get blind-sided, and I think most PWPs would agree with me.

Because I continued to be concerned about ongoing mental "fogginess," I discussed it with Dr. Kluger. Though the atrophy question had been removed, I was still concerned about the aMCI diagnosis and its possible implications. I am sure that anxiety was still an issue as well. In any case, Dr. Kluger recommended that I start taking Aricept. I interpreted this as a precautionary measure that might help with symptoms and/or slow progression if, in fact, I was progressing toward dementia. With subjects like this, Dr. Kluger would sometimes be somewhat vague, I think to avoid raising my anxiety level further. Based on our conversations and how much I knew (or at least thought I knew) on these subjects, I am sure he was abundantly aware of my anxiety level in spite of the calm demeanor I typically try to project.

From the start, I wrestled with how much I wanted to share with Linda, my sons, relatives, and friends. Early on I decided that I would be open about it. After all, I would want to know if the proverbial shoe were on the other foot. On the one hand, I think it is a good thing for family and friends to be concerned and praying for each other. On the other hand, while I want them to be informed, I don't want to have them overly concerned or feeling sorry for me. This is a conundrum and a fine line to walk for most PD patients, I think. It is sometimes difficult to determine how much information is enough and how much is too much. This is complicated by the fact that different people receive information like this in different ways. Some are very caring, accepting, and compassionate. Some put up mental "force fields" and seem to want to question the validity of what you are telling them or just avoid the subject altogether. All I can do is attempt to communicate what I would want them to tell me if the situation were reversed. However, I have noticed that some people need time to process these things and become more open later on.

In late January, our older son and his wife sold their house after having it on the market for only a week (almost miraculous given how slow the real estate market was at that point). As part of our financial strategizing, we had begun thinking about selling our current large home and moving closer to our kids (who were at that point about a 45-minute drive north) and our five (soon to be six) grandchildren. It was clear that we would eventually want to downsize and, with all the grandkids, our kids could certainly use our help. However, it was a tough decision to leave the beautiful place that had been our dream home since we moved to Colorado. We investigated a lot of options for a move and did a lot of praying, but I must say we were encouraged by our son's success in selling his place so quickly (and for a fair price). We made our decision to take the plunge and put the house on the market, which had been extremely soft since the onset of the financial institution crisis the previous fall. We listed the house in early June 2009 and, to our surprise, had a contract signed within a week (pretty much identical to what had happened with our son's house only a few months earlier). We threw our house hunt into high gear and decided on a maintenance-free patio home in a 55+ community close to both of our sons, which had come on the market the previous fall. We thought it would be a good fit for us, but never expected it to be available when we were ready to buy! It was about half the size of our previous house, which is what we wanted, but very nice. Miraculously, we were also able to obtain a low-interest mortgage. We lined up a mover, and ended up closing on our old place one day in early July, closing on the new place the next morning, and moving in that afternoon!

At this point, Linda and I were stunned by our good fortune. So many pieces had fallen into place in the past year that enabled us to make this move, maintain a reasonable level of financial security, and keep our sanity, in spite of my illness. We believed that God had richly blessed us once again and we were thankful! Because we had been able to move so much faster than we estimated, Linda would have an hour-long commute to work each day, but she was OK with that as our plan was for her to retire in about six months. The only really big remaining piece was that I had not yet received SSDI approval, which would provide critical financial security as well as early Medicare coverage.

Shortly after we moved, I was extremely disappointed to receive a letter from Social Security informing me that my disability application had been rejected. I had to consider the possibility of re-entering the job market, but knew there was not much I could do. I couldn't see myself doing anything much more challenging than being a greeter at Walmart (no offense to Walmart greeters intended), but knew that fatigue and acuity would make even that a problem! Stress, my biggest enemy, roared back with a vengeance.

I had been told that an SSDI denial was likely to happen, but I had really believed it wouldn't. I knew that it was possible to appeal the rejection, but didn't know how to go about it, what it would cost, how long it would take, what the likelihood of success was, or any other details. Characteristically, I immediately set out to learn all I could in this area. I was referred to a respected attorney who specializes in these matters and set up a meeting. I was encouraged when she concluded that she thought I should have been approved and that, with her firm carrying the ball, she thought I would be approved upon resubmission, though of course she could offer no guarantees. It seems that Social Security's standard operating procedure is to reject first applications in anything other than black-and-white situations that met all their policies and criteria. The cost of pursuing an appeal was reasonable, all things considered (there would be no fee if I was not approved), but the process could take up to a year. If I were to be approved, benefits would be paid retroactive to my qualification date, which I had submitted as September 2008, the month after I was unable to continue working. In conjunction with that, I would qualify for Medicare in February 2011, a few months after my 62nd birthday. So, once again, it was "leap of faith" time, and I signed on the dotted line.

Late in 2009, I decided to try to direct some of my energy to the needs of others. That month, I wrote an article in our new senior community's newsletter about a meeting to be held at my house for people who were interested in participating in a community Parkinson's support group. I had already met a couple of neighbors who had PD and quickly heard about others. We currently have 15 active members (including caregivers). Many of us are also active in the Highlands Ranch support group and are members of the Parkinson's Association of the Rockies (PAR).

The fears I was dealing with are not surprising in light of current medical knowledge and thinking. The importance of non-motor symptoms (cognition, depression, anxiety, dementia, sleep issues, and more) has been a hot topic in the medical community at least since the beginning of 2010. In the foreword of *Parkinson Disease: Mind, Mood, & Memory* (National Parkinson Foundation), Dr. Matthew Stern (Director, Parkinson's Disease and Movement Disorder at Pennsylvania Hospital) wrote that "it is the neurobehavioral aspects of PD that frequently define a patient's true sense of well-being. We now realize that while tremor, stiffness and slowness are clinical hallmarks of PD, it is 'mind, mood and memory' that really matter."

Chapter 6: Deep Brain Stimulation

During the latter part of 2009, I decided to make an appointment at one of the top neurological hospitals in the United States. I was not dissatisfied with the University of Colorado Hospital (UCH),[19] but thought it was a good idea to pursue another expert opinion. I had a number of options where friends or family lived in the vicinity of the target hospital. Barrow Neurological Institute[20] (also home to the Muhammad Ali Parkinson Clinic) in Phoenix offered to make an appointment with me and I accepted (I have friends who live in Sun City West, which is in the area). I was happy to learn that I would be meeting with Dr. Abraham Lieberman, an internationally recognized PD expert, former medical director at the National Parkinson Foundation (NPF), and director of both Barrows and the Ali Clinic.

I met with Dr. Lieberman during November of 2009. During his in-depth examination, he commented that I would be an excellent candidate for deep brain stimulation (DBS) surgery. He mentioned that DBS was highly successful in addressing tremor, which was clearly my most troublesome motor symptom. He recommended trying some different medications to see if there might be a nonsurgical solution. He also told me that he had met the team at UCH and that he felt they were an excellent choice if I decided to pursue DBS surgery.

When I returned to Denver, I spoke to Dr. Kluger about my visit at Barrow. He agreed that I would be a good DBS candidate if a medication could not be found that solved the problem (he knew my case well enough that he did not think this was likely). After trying a number of medications that didn't help, I made an appointment for a DBS evaluation.

The first step in the evaluation was another neuropsychological exam, which I took in December 2009. As I understand it, they do not do DBS in cases where there is evidence of dementia. I had the same neuropsychologist for this exam. As I have already mentioned, he interpreted the results as showing that there was no longer evidence of mild cognitive impairment

(MCI) and I was approved from a neuropsychological standpoint based on this test.

The next step in the process, which took place in April 2010, was an in-depth PD exam by a movement disorder specialist while I was taking Sinemet.[21] The next day I was examined after having been off Sinemet overnight. Unified Parkinson Disease Rating Scale (UPDRS)[22] scores are compared both on and off Sinemet. If functioning is not significantly worse off Sinemet, approval is not likely, as this differential correlates positively to the likelihood that DBS will be effective. I was also evaluated by a specialist to determine if I was likely to need voice therapy. Finally, I met with the neurosurgeon, Dr. Steven Ojemann, who made sure that I was aware of the risks and benefits associated with DBS. After some discussion, we agreed that the logical target for my DBS would be the thalamus,[23] which he described as the best target for tremor (the target for general PD symptoms is usually the subthalamic nucleus[24] or globus pallidus). About a week later, I was told that I had been approved. I could have scheduled the surgery at that time, but had to wait for insurance reasons—needless to say, insurance coverage was an important aspect of this decision. We set a tentative surgery date for March 2011.

In hindsight, it was good that we waited because it gave us a chance to do our homework and get additional feedback. For example, in July 2010 my wife and I traveled to Bethesda, Maryland, to participate in a National Institute of Health/ National Institute of Neurological Disease & Stroke (NIH/ NINDS)[25] clinical research program for development of a PD patient database. While there, I learned a good deal more about the disease and some things specific to me (such as that my sense of smell was significantly diminished). I also took the opportunity to ask about DBS and whether there was something else on the horizon research-wise that I should wait for. The NINDS personnel spoke highly of UCH, agreed with the thalamus target based on their exam, and told me that DBS was my best option for the foreseeable future. This added to our confidence that we were on the right track.

Another benefit of waiting was that we started attending Bionic Brigade[26] DBS support group meetings in our area. This gave us the opportunity to learn more about DBS surgery and life after DBS directly from patients. The bottom line is that, for most PD patients, there is a window of opportunity when they can take advantage of procedures that will improve their quality of life. That window is finite. While I didn't hear anyone say that

DBS is perfect, I also did not hear anyone say that they would not do it over again. My wife and I were armed with enough information to decide to take the plunge.

March 2011 finally arrived. I was to have three surgeries; the first two would involve implantation of the leads from both sides of my brain into the thalamus. Extensions would be connected to the leads and run under my scalp, where they would later be connected to the neurostimulator[27] that would be implanted in my upper left chest (the third surgery).

I was given antibiotic ointment that was applied with a Q-Tip in the nose for a week prior to surgery, as well as a special shampoo for my hair. This was to minimize the risk of infection, one the most common DBS issues. CT scans were taken before and after each of the first two surgeries. The first helped determine the trajectory for implantation of the lead. The second ensured that the placement was correct and that there were no apparent problems. The first two surgeries were inpatient and included an overnight stay in the neurology ICU where I would be observed and helped with any problems. One of the least pleasant memories of the surgery was the placement of the "halo" that would stabilize my head during surgery. A local anesthetic was used to minimize discomfort, but the pressure from the halo was uncomfortable. The halo was rendered immobile with four screws that were attached to my skull (there was no pain with this, but the idea was gruesome). Without this device, DBS would not be possible, as it holds the head completely still during surgery. I was sedated for surgery, but it had been explained to me that I would be conscious for part of the surgery so that I could give feedback that would help ensure proper placement of the leads.

The primary players in the operating room were the neurosurgeon, the movement disorder neurologist, and the Medtronic[28] representative (Medtronic is a medical technology company that manufactures DBS components, works with doctors and neurosurgeons, and is involved in DBS surgeries). I was aware that all three were involved in the discussions and decision making, though the neurosurgeon made the final call when necessary. For each of these first two surgeries, the movement disorder neurologist had me write my name, draw a straight line, and draw a circular pattern both before and during surgery. It was amazing to see how steady I was in the operating room compared to my preliminary drawings. When Linda saw these drawings, she was astounded. I was also asked whether I felt anything unusual, like numbness or tingling, when adjustments were made to the lead placement. There was no pain associated with this (the brain does not feel pain). I was not awake at the beginning of the operation, so thankfully missed the drilling of the holes in my skull.

The first two surgeries were a week apart. The third, which was an outpatient procedure for implantation of the neurostimulator (about the size of a small cell phone), was two weeks later. I was under general anesthesia for this one. The extensions run from the leads to a point in the back of the head (under the scalp) where they are connected; from there, a single extension runs behind my left ear down my neck and across my collarbone where it connects to the neurostimulator.

The neurostimulator is not turned on for about two weeks following the last surgery, to allow initial healing to take place. At that time, I had my first "programming" session with the physician assistant, who adjusted the settings of the neurostimulator to provide the maximum benefit with the fewest side effects. In my case, if the settings are too strong, it affects my face and jaw muscles and makes it difficult to speak clearly. Over the course of four visits, we were able to fine-tune the settings. I was pleased that my "programmer" (rather like a remote control) has four programs within which I can adjust the stimulation level up or down on both sides of my brain.

Besides programming, postsurgery issues include following the regimen to minimize the chance of infection, allowing the wounds to heal, getting used to managing the neurostimulator, and avoiding exposure to magnetic devices (including MRIs). Now I always opt out of going through any scanning devices. I would prefer not to have to do this, but the manual procedure is not that bad once you get used to it. It takes a little while to get used to having the device in your chest, but it is very much the same as the pacemaker that many people have for heart conditions. In fact, I often describe DBS as a "pacemaker for the brain." Having the implant has also ended my dreams of being a swimsuit model, but that is a sacrifice I am willing to make.

I have experienced numerous benefits from the surgery. My hand tremor only shows up intermittently now, and only in stressful situations. I have no head tremor at all. I appreciate that I am no longer stared at in restaurants. Plus I am now able to putt (I used to be a pretty good golfer) and chip (the tremor affected my short game more than anything else) without shaking. Serving a tennis ball, which used to be a joke (who knew where the ball was going to go when I tossed it?), is now doable, though I can't run around the court like I used to due to slowness and potential for falls. But I'm not complaining. I can do things I enjoy, and, best of all, have fun playing with my grandchildren.

The memory of these surgeries is fading, but the benefit is not. I would always urge anyone considering DBS surgery to ask a lot of questions. At the end of the day, it is up to you to decide whether DBS is right for you. My feeling was that I wanted to take advantage of a procedure that would improve my quality of life if the benefits outweighed the risks. I am glad that I had DBS and would do it again.

However, there is one particular concern that I hope will receive attention in the future. In chapter 12, "Grace" mentions in her interview that her mother, who at that time had been diagnosed with dementia, but not Lewy body dementia, was "never the same" following a mastectomy surgery. It was Grace's feeling that this deterioration was caused by the surgery. In hindsight, I wonder if my DBS surgeries or the anesthesia used in March/April 2011 may have exacerbated an undiagnosed problem that I had been experiencing since 2008. Specifically, I experienced significant cognitive issues, including difficulty thinking clearly and communicating, following both lead-implant surgeries. I have since learned that the side effects of surgery is an area of concern to the medical community. Once again, I bear no ill will toward anyone at my hospital, especially since this hypothesis may be inaccurate. I am confident that I received the best possible treatment and advice based on what was known at that time. I hope that there will be further research regarding the potential dangers of surgery and anesthesia in connection with LBD.

Chapter 7: Bad News/Good News

During September 2011, five months after my successful deep brain stimulation surgery, I took the Montreal Cognitive Assessment,[29] a short version of a neuropsych evaluation, due to a recurrence of cognition problems. The results indicated a sufficient level of memory problems for Dr. Kluger to recommend that I start using the Exelon patch, a medication used for mild to moderate Alzheimer's disease or Parkinson's dementia. It seemed to me that "the patch" did help (more some days than others), but my memory problems got worse by the next summer, leading Dr. Kluger to have me take my third "neuropsych" in July 2012. While most of my brain functioning was normal or better (in some cases much better) with no indication of an underlying dementia, the neuropsychologist reported that the results were consistent with amnestic mild cognitive impairment (aMCI). For me it was déjà vu all over again.

In early 2011, I wrote a PD-related children's book, *Carson and His Shaky Paws Grampa*, with illustrations by fellow PWP, Alison Paolini. I created a Shaky Paws Facebook page for the book and a Shaky Paws Grampa blog that I have used to post articles about my writing and advocacy work, information related to PD and cognition issues, and living with PD and cognitive challenges. I am amazed to report that my blog and Facebook page have been visited by people in the United States, Russia, Germany, UK, Ukraine, France, Canada, Latvia, Australia, Israel, Romania, Pakistan, Portugal, Ireland, Vietnam, South Korea, Saudi Arabia, Ecuador, Malaysia, India, Belarus, Georgia, Indonesia, China, Denmark, Sweden, Netherlands, Cayman Islands, Seychelles, Bolivia, Poland, Italy, Egypt, United Arab Emirates, Brazil, Bulgaria, Venezuela, Argentina, Serbia, Netherlands, Greece, Romania, Philippines, and Jamaica.

After the *Carson* book was published, I had the opportunity to speak at a variety of support group meetings and "Meet the Doctor" seminars to talk about my personal experience with PD, DBS, and the book. I did a 15-minute radio interview regarding these subjects in December 2011. In early February 2012, while in Phoenix to speak to support groups at the Muhammad Ali PD Center, I was interviewed by Fox TV as part of a feature on PD. An article on my book, Carson, and me appeared in the Sunday *Denver Post* book review section on February 26, 2012. On April 11, 2012, I was the keynote speaker at the Parkinson Association of the Rockies (PAR) "Triumph" fundraiser event.

I applied (on behalf of both Linda and myself) to the Parkinson Disease Foundation (PDF) in hopes of being selected to attend a Clinical Research Learning Institute training session for the western United States to be held in California during July 2012. We were chosen, completed the training, and in the process met the dedicated PDF staff; doctors involved in various aspects of the research process; and many interesting, involved, and knowledgeable fellow research advocates. We are now involved in presentations regarding the importance of participation in research as part of PDF's Parkinson's Advocates in Research (PAIR) program to support groups.

I had a second children's book, *Carina and Her Care Partner Gramma*, published during September 2013. Linda and I are involved in three support groups (a new group for PWPs with cognitive issues and their care partners, a local PD support group, and the Bionic Brigade) and actively participate as members of the Parkinson Association of the Rockies.

Linda and I attended the third World Parkinson Congress (WPC) in Montreal, held during the first week of October 2013. We had the honor of being chosen to be among the first patient participants in the PDF's Parkinson Study Group meetings. We were able to interact and share ideas for research with two of the working groups (neurosurgery and cognitive/psychiatric), which are composed of doctors and research scientists from all over the world. We attended many presentations by elite international PD organizations and individuals regarding important PD developments. I was very encouraged by research being done involving alpha-synuclein,[30] a protein that seems to play a key role in the formation of the Lewy bodies[31] that are associated with PD and Lewy body dementia. I was also pleased about the amount of attention being paid to patient involvement/ engagement in the medical and research community, which acknowledges the important role patients and their families can play.

I was extraordinarily energized when we returned to our home following the WPC. Linda and I have been able to share our experience and what we learned with the PD community here, as well as around the world (via my blog). Most importantly, I carried back with me a kind of "glow" based on a strong sense of love and community that was created by all who attended. It is something I have felt whenever I interact with other PWPs, caregivers, or individuals in PD support organizations—an atmosphere of mutual caring, camaraderie, and acceptance. It was at that point that I added the rainbow to the cover for this book.

Chapter 8: Parkinson's and Dementia

I have had many opportunities to speak with other PD patients through support groups, conferences, advocacy presentations, individual meetings, and just talking with friends. Without question, a significant concern for most patients (perhaps less so with young-onset PD[32]) is whether they will end up with dementia. Their concern is not surprising, since most PWPs feel the effects of bradyphrenia[33] (slowness in mental processing due to a decreased ability to shift quickly from one conceptual pattern to another; most often seen with PD) and wonder if their mental status will get worse. PWPs and care partners should definitely discuss any concerns about cognition or memory with their movement disorder specialist (MDS). The MDS will help determine the most likely cause(s) of the problems, which can include depression, side effects from other medications, vitamin B12 deficiency, and others.

According to the Mayo Clinic, *dementia* is not a specific disease. "Instead, dementia describes a group of symptoms affecting thinking and social abilities severely enough to interfere with daily functioning." The two types of dementia most frequently associated with PD are Parkinson's disease dementia[34] (PDD) and Lewy body dementia[35] (LBD). Detailed information on these conditions, including diagnostic criteria, appears in appendix A at the end of this book. The diagnostic process for both of these conditions is similar[36]; in fact, there is some debate as to whether these are actually different illnesses or the same disease with different manifestations. The primary distinction between the two is time of onset: LBD is diagnosed if the dementia symptoms start before, concurrent with, or slightly after onset of PD motor symptoms. PDD is the diagnosis when the dementia symptoms occur years after the onset of motor symptoms.

There are, however, key differences between Lewy body dementia and Alzheimer's (technically known as "dementia of the Alzheimer's type")[37]:

- **Memory loss** tends to be a more prominent symptom in early Alzheimer's than in early LBD, although advanced LBD may cause memory problems in addition to its more typical effects on judgment, planning, and visual perception.

- **Movement symptoms** are more likely to be an important cause of disability early in LBD than in Alzheimer's, although Alzheimer's can cause problems with walking, balance, and getting around as it progresses to moderate and severe stages.

- **Hallucinations**, delusions, and misidentification of familiar people are significantly more frequent in early-stage LBD than in Alzheimer's.

- **REM sleep disorder** is more common in early LBD than in Alzheimer's.

- **Disruption of the autonomic nervous system,** causing a blood pressure drop on standing, dizziness, falls, and urinary incontinence, is much more common in early LBD than in Alzheimer's.

Many PWPs experience problems with word finding, attention, organization, scheduling, planning, mental inflexibility (decrease in neuroplasticity[38]), multitasking, recall of verbal information, spatial disorientation, hallucinations, interruption of "train of thought," and possibly other areas of mental functioning. Some of these abilities fall into categories called *executive function*[39] and *working memory.*[40] Typical estimates in the past for the percentage of PD patients with dementia at any point in time are about 40%, though this number is subject to debate. A 2010 Cambridge research paper[41] states: "As Parkinson's disease dementia has been associated with mortality, longitudinal estimates of its cumulative prevalence, rather than cross-section estimates, are more accurate representations of true dementia frequency within the Parkinson's disease population, and range from 75% to 90%." This reflects the fact that dementia is a common development in the later stages of PD. According to Dr. Kluger, these studies were of people with Parkinson's disease for 20 years or longer and included mainly elderly subjects. It is likely that younger people with PD have a lower risk. It should also be noted that these studies started 20 years ago and that advances in treatment and promotion of exercise may also lower this risk. The level of longitudinal frequency remains a subject of debate.

Some doctors are reluctant to talk openly about this subject due to legitimate concerns about patient reaction. However, if it is important to PWPs to know as much as possible about all aspects of their current condition so that they can participate in decision making and make informed choices for their future, they may want to be insistent. It is important to understand that doctors may not always be able to provide answers for questions, even if they would like to. If PWPs have symptoms that concern them and other causes have been ruled out, they can ask if the doctor will administer the Montreal Cognitive Assessment, a test that can be done in the doctor's office in about 15 minutes. This provides the doctor with a "snapshot" of the PWP's current condition in potential problem areas related to PD, including mild cognitive impairment.[42] The best way to get the most reliable feedback is to take a full neuropsychological assessment[43] administered by a neuropsychologist. PWPs should be able to get a referral from their doctor if the doctor agrees that it is appropriate.

The main reason that there has been reluctance to discuss dementia openly, I think, is that Alzheimer's, Parkinson's dementia. and Lewy body dementia are all terminal conditions. Also, most of us find the possibility of being unable to communicate or even recognize those we love to be extremely frightening. Dementia Guide.com states that for PDD and LBD, "the duration of either disease is 'several years' from onset of symptoms." In contrast, the Lewy Body Disease Association (which includes both diseases under the LBD "umbrella") states that "the disease has an average duration of 5 to 7 years. It is possible, though, for the time span to be anywhere from 2 to 20 years, depending on several factors, including the person's overall health, age and severity of symptoms." This disparity in information can't help but create confusion and anxiety for patients, caregivers, and families.

A statement that PWPs often hear is that people don't die as a direct result of PD, but rather from other conditions that develop along with it. One of the most frequent causes of death that is a direct result of PD is aspiration pneumonia, caused by swallowing problems. However, with current research telling us that a significant majority of PWPs develop life-ending dementia that is clearly related to PD, it seems incongruous to say that PD is not a cause of death. Once again, I think that this is done to reduce fear and anxiety in PWPs and their families.

The following is an encouraging excerpt from a Fox blog post, dated January 21, 2013, regarding a joint clinical trial being undertaken by the Michael J. Fox Foundation and Sanofi Pharmaceuticals for a drug to treat PD-related cognitive decline:

This is important, because, while cognitive dysfunction is a troublesome reality for many people living with Parkinson's, it is not well-understood. Symptoms can range from slowness of thinking or difficulty organizing and sequencing one's thoughts, to memory loss, to the eventual onset of dementia. The only approved therapy currently on the market for PD dementia is the Exelon Patch (rivastigmine) which only modestly improves symptoms. An overriding hurdle to drug development for cognitive decline is that little is known about the underlying disease processes taking place in the brain.[44]

The cost of any neurodegenerative disease to patients, caregivers, families, and society has been well documented. Obviously, we are talking about emotional impact as well as financial. The University of Pennsylvania Perelman School of Medicine[45] published information describing the size of the problem relating to the volume and cost of brain diseases and injuries. The current cost was estimated to be about $600 billion per year. For Alzheimer's alone, the American Health Assistance Foundation[46] states that "over 5 million (5.4 million) Americans age 65 and older are thought to have Alzheimer's disease. By 2050, the number of Americans with this disease could increase to over 15 million. The national cost of Alzheimer's disease (in people over 65 years old) was $183 billion in 2011, and by 2050 it will be $1.1 trillion." Without question, the size of the problem is enormous.

The importance of this issue was made apparent by the announcement, on April 2, 2013, of a new research program called the BRAIN (Brain Research through Advancing Innovative Neurotechnologies) Initiative. This is an exciting development for people with neurodegenerative diseases, as the BRAIN program will link research supported by the Defense Advanced Research Projects Agency, the National Institutes of Health, and the National Science Foundation. "This new public-private partnership initiative offers a great opportunity to accelerate the support of research that can lead to breakthroughs for the treatment and ultimately prevention and cure of mental illness," said Jeffrey Borenstein, MD, editor-in-chief of *Psychiatric News* and president of the Brain and Behavior Research Foundation.[47]

The seriousness of this problem is fueling a close examination of current practices in palliative care and hospice, which I discuss in chapter 13.

Chapter 9: Stress

A 2011 article on the *Scientific American* website, titled "Neurostress: How Stress May Fuel Neurodegenerative Diseases,"[48] discusses stress as a causative factor of disease, including PD. My personal opinion is that stress in all its forms deserves more attention.

Clearly, stress is part of our everyday lives at work or play. Not all stress is bad. However, based on the personality, tolerance level, and genetic background of individuals, stress can create cellular oxidative stress[49] and inflammation[50] that have been linked to many different types of diseases, including the neurodegenerative variety; possible causative factors include cell damage and toxicity. A 2012 paper published on the Intech website[51] provides a good (though somewhat complicated) explanation.

We have been hearing for a long time about the dangers of free radicals and the benefits of antioxidants.[52] *Free radicals* are chemically reactive molecules released when cells are damaged by oxidative stress, inflammation, or other factors. Free radicals attack healthy cells, injuring them and increasing the potential for disease. Antioxidants are the body's defense against free radicals; they are found in various types of foods, especially fruits, vegetables, and whole grains. I am not going to recommend a particular strategy for supplementing the body's natural ability to produce antioxidants. This is a subject that patients can discuss with their doctors. I would, however, like to call attention to genetic factors that vary among individuals and are, in my opinion, worth knowing about.

Information regarding genetic risk factors related to Alzheimer's is available on the National Institute of Health's National Institute on Aging website,[53] which states:

> Increased risk is related to the apolipoprotein E (APOE) gene found on chromosome 19. APOE contains the instructions for making a protein that helps carry cholesterol and other types of fat in the bloodstream. APOE comes in several different forms, or alleles. Three

forms—APOE ε2, APOE ε3, and APOE ε4—occur most frequently.

APOE ε2 is relatively rare and may provide some protection against the disease. If Alzheimer's disease occurs in a person with this allele, it develops later in life than it would in someone with the APOE ε4 gene.

APOE ε3, the most common allele, is believed to play a neutral role in the disease—neither decreasing nor increasing risk.

APOE ε4 is present in about 25 to 30 percent of the population and in about 40 percent of all people with late-onset Alzheimer's. People who develop Alzheimer's are more likely to have an APOE ε4 allele than people who do not develop the disease.

If you have a family history of neurodegenerative disease, it may be a good idea to find out if you have the APOE4 gene from both parents. Testing is currently available but not routine. It is likely to be much more accessible in the future. If you are at risk, you have the opportunity to be proactive by adjusting your lifestyle, diet, and make other changes to reduce the risk of developing the disease, as well as obtaining treatment to improve quality of life.

Other potential sources of stress we all live with may include:

- Anything ingested into the body, including water, other liquids, and food
- The air we breathe
- Smoking (ironically, current research has shown that nicotine reduces the risk of PD)
- Pollution
- Life/work/relationships
- Psychological factors related to Maslow's hierarchy of human needs[54] (poor self-esteem, for example)
- Exposure to or ingestion of toxins, including pesticides (not sure if alcohol should be included in this category, but it seems likely, especially when consumed excessively)
- Excess weight
- Overall health

So, life as we know it can increase our chances of developing any number of diseases. Each of us has the opportunity to learn as much as we can to enable us to make informed choices for safeguarding our own health as well as the health of our families. Or we can choose to not know and just hope for the best (a position that is understandable, though I don't subscribe to it), which I know is the preference of some.

It seems important to consider what factors contribute to symptoms related to various conditions and, more importantly, the root causes behind these problems. Perhaps at some point we will decide to examine our priorities as individuals, couples, and families and make some tough decisions regarding wants vs. needs, what we do for a living, where we live, what we eat and drink, how we relax, and more. It is natural to be lulled into complacency by a sense that we do not have choices. The truth is that for most of us, society, our neighbors, our friends, TV advertising, and more establish the constraints we choose to live within. The trend today for many is toward a fast-paced, complicated life where acquisition and thrill seeking are the priorities. Technology is a good thing for the most part, but when we become slaves to communication (social networking, email, texting, cell phones, and more), we may need to call for a time out to rethink things. How we choose to spend our time, energy, and resources is always going to be subject to change based on new developments. Regardless, there will always be a need for balance and perspective. These are my opinions, for what they are worth.

I have not always been this erudite. It is something I have acquired over time, much as a ship acquires barnacles. I have experienced stress in relationships, most notably with my father, and in a career that, although it included success and accomplishment, was marked by frequent changes and disappointment due to career dissonance[55] (caused by disparity between a person's gifts and his or her career choices).

I have worked with a tool called the Myers Briggs Type Indicator [56] (MBTI) over the years to build my own self-awareness and to assist others in making career and life choices. I am particularly passionate about providing teenagers with self-awareness tools, as a means of gaining appreciation for the importance and opportunity connected with taking ownership of their lives. Life is full of unexpected developments, and these tools can help create a "template" that can be used to make informed choices over the course of a lifetime.

In MBTI-speak, I am a clear INFJ.[57] More than 60 years of research has shown INFJs to be inspirational, visionary, empathetic, insightful leaders (their ranks include people like Nelson Mandela and Mother Teresa); however, they also have a propensity to internalize problems and tend to take on a disproportionate degree of responsibility. While I would in no way compare myself to the aforementioned individuals in terms of accomplishments, I believe that we do share some common traits.

I would encourage further research (I know there has been some) to study the impact of dissonance between an individual's "type" (using the Myers Briggs Type Indicator or something similar) and their life choices on stress levels and psychological wellness.

I understand that any individual's ability to cope with stressful life events and situations is a function of a variety of variables, not least of which is the person's innate ability to let problems "roll off their back" based on their personalities. There are a variety of coping strategies, including meditation, squeezing a rubber ball, chopping wood, and alcoholism (not recommended), but I believe it is far more desirable to identify and proactively address root causes, as mentioned earlier.

Perhaps Thoreau[58] was onto something with his focus on a simple, uncomplicated life. It is not realistic to think that we can control all the stress-creating factors in our lives. But if we identify those things that we *can* control, make a few adjustments to our priorities, add a few healthy stress management techniques and some self-awareness tools, maybe we can nudge the scales in a direction that will reduce stress and create better balance.

Chapter 10: Living with Parkinson's
and Cognitive Impairment

Since I am committed to being open on this subject, I will describe this intermediate stage between "normal" cognition and dementia—amnestic mild cognitive impairment (aMCI)—including what it feels like and what I am experiencing. There is no definitive test that confirms PD-related dementia (except autopsy, which I think would be premature), so it is to a large extent up to me to determine the significance, if any, of these experiences.

It should be noted that some of what I am experiencing could be attributed to PD medications, PD in general, or the normal aging process as opposed to aMCI, but this seems difficult to pinpoint. With that in mind, I will provide "effect" information and leave it to others to try to determine cause. For example, fatigue is experienced by roughly 50% of PD patients, whereas a symptom of dementia can be excessive daytime sleepiness, a more persistent form of fatigue not attributable to lack of normal sleep. Also, vivid dreams have been associated with some PD meds, and are also associated with the REM sleep disorders commonly seen with Lewy body dementia.

- My dreams for the past four years have often been unusual, and have included scary incidents where I am attacked by animals or people and wake up fighting them off; vivid dreams that feel psychotic; and dreams that feel like those we have all had when we have a fever. Linda woke me up recently because I was having a scary dream and making loud noises. I was in a car that had, for no reason, become filled with small bugs. In addition, there were some large abstract bug-like creatures on the dashboard. I was able to pick up some of these and throw them out the car window. However, one vigorously resisted being thrown out. I managed to get it out and started driving away. Whatever this "thing" was kept pace outside my window as I accelerated, so I closed the window just in time to keep it out. At this point, I was scared. To my horror (a strong word, but that is what it was), this "thing," now joined by many identical creatures, got hold of the top of the window and began to open it. I was yelling in my dream when Linda woke me up. This was not the first time that I have been afraid to go back to sleep.

- I frequently forget things (like glasses or my meds) when leaving the house. I usually remember and go back to get them. I have lost an assortment of water bottles, sunglasses, reading glasses, and even clothes. I was on a trip and went into the bathroom at a gas station to take off the sweat pants I had been wearing over a pair of shorts because it had been cold earlier. Unfortunately, I left the sweat pants hanging in the stall when I exited and didn't remember them until we were well down the road.

- About a year ago I started to experience what I call "short circuits" when talking that momentarily make it difficult to speak. They have become more frequent recently and usually seem to be related to stress.

- I sometimes find loud noise (especially in an otherwise quiet setting) to be painful. This seems to happen most when I am tired. I have also noticed that I am easily startled—so much so that if someone plays a joke on me (like most of us do) to scare me, they get an unexpected reaction (which I describe as the "upside-down-cat-with-its-claws-embedded-in-the-ceiling" syndrome). On a related note (I think), I am sensitive to bright light. I notice this when riding in a car and driving under a tree when there is bright sunlight. The intermittent flashes of bright light going in and out of the shade are actually painful. Another example of this occurred when I had retina laser surgery to repair minor tears and a detachment. Between the laser bursts that repaired these problems and the extremely bright light used to examine the work being done, I was in agony. I know this is not the case with "normal" patients who have an intact nervous system.

- Multi-tasking is a problem for me, as it is for many with PD. The first time I realized this was when I tried to sing and clap my hands at the same time, something I had always been able to do. Another example was at a physical therapy evaluation when the therapist had me try to walk and count backward from 100 subtracting 7 each time. Yikes!

- I function best within the structure of routines. This summer we took a car trip with my sister and brother-in-law up to Canmore, Alberta (Canada), to spend time in the Canadian Rockies. I had a great time, but was glad to return to my own bed and familiar routines.

- I get tired easily, especially following periods of concentration (like working on the computer) or heightened attention (such as those few occasions when I drive), and take at least one nap daily.

- If I overdo it on any particular day (physically or mentally), I usually need more down time the next day to recover. I have found that a mind-over-matter approach does not work. It is important for me to find balance between my level of engagement and the rest I need.

- I have difficulty keeping track of planned events and appointments without the help of my wife, reminder lists, and our appointment book. Even with these assists, I often forget things I was supposed to do. For example, the Parkinson Disease Foundation (PDF) schedules national calls with its research associates (which include Linda and me). I have missed these calls two months in a row, the first due to failure to take into account the time difference. Linda was not home for the January call (due to babysitting sick grandkids) and I missed it in spite of the fact that it was in our schedule book. I remembered later that night.

- I have trouble with tasks that are complex in nature. My wife has taken over most matters related to preparation of our tax files for our accountant, a job that I handled routinely in the past. I bought a laptop computer last year and was intimidated by the setup process. So it remained unused for about six months until my brother-in-law helped me with it.

- I sometimes remember things at night that I couldn't during the day. I assume that this is because there is very little competing mental "traffic" at that time. I sometimes get up and write down ideas so that I will be able to go back to sleep. I recently purchased a small voice recorder that I plan to keep on my nightstand to make this easier.

- My dear wife and care partner will confirm that if I don't get the rest I need, I am prone to becoming crabby, at which point she will invite me to go take a nap. At least we both recognize this now and can deal with it. In the past, I would subject her to angry outbursts or "robust criticism" that left both of us feeling bad, almost always when I was overtired. I am not the kind of person who likes to hurt anyone, least of all her.

- Another problem I am trying to deal with is mood swings. I have pronounced ups and downs, which I am able to manage only up to a point. I find that the antidepressant I take daily helps, and see this as a useful part of my medication regimen rather than as a sign of weakness.

- I believe that my level of commitment to some projects or activities over the past couple of years could be viewed as obsessive/compulsive. Linda often points this out in terms of the amount of time I spend on the computer. A more concrete example of this is that, when getting ready for bed, if I splash some water on the countertop by our sinks, I am unable to *not* wipe it up.

- I have experienced a burst of creativity for the past month. I believe it started after Linda and I traveled to Manhattan, where the golden years of my career took place, to be the subject of a Medtronic DBS photo shoot. This was in addition to the Christmas season, which always lifts my spirits. But my excitement rose to a new level when my younger son, Brian, and his family returned from China (where they had been living since

July) a few days later for the holidays. Since then I have finished my second children's book, which was published in September 2013; am pursuing an ambitious music project to benefit PD; and have finished this book, which has been a dream of mine for at least four years.

- I get confused much more easily and take longer to process information needed to make decisions. For example, I went to the store recently to pick up something for a quick dinner for my grandchildren when their mom was sick. I thought fried chicken and sides would be easy. However, when I saw all the varieties of fried chicken (nuggets, fingers, wings, á la carte options, and dinner combinations), as well as multiple sides, it took way more time than it should have to decide what to get. The gentleman attempting to serve me clearly could sense that I was struggling, though I tried to maintain a nonchalant demeanor. Fortunately, when I stopped at the Redbox to pick up a movie, the latest "Diary of a Wimpy Kid" movie was on the first line, making a potentially laborious evaluation process quick and easy.

- I use a timer to help me remember to take my pills. If my timer goes off, I have to take the pill right away or I will forget, usually remembering up to an hour or more after that because I feel crummy from not taking the pill. I carry my timer and a pill supply wherever I go.

- I have been describing the way I experience time (for about the past year) as "ethereal." That is the best word I can come up with. Time just doesn't seem as finite as it used to. Periods of time go by inordinately quickly. In addition, it is sometimes difficult for me to remember what I did during those periods of time.

- Sometimes when I wake up, it feels like I am still asleep, even though I know I'm not. I can't help but feel that, at some point in the future, the lines between sleep and wakefulness will become increasingly blurred.

I will admit that I have experienced some anxiety over these developments, because I know that some of them are indications that my cognition issues are progressing. However, over time, Linda and I have chosen not to dwell on them or take them too seriously. We even laugh sometimes when I do something silly, which is more often some days than others. What will happen is out of my hands, so I focus on making choices that I feel good about and that will enable us to enjoy our lives together.

Chapter 11: Choices

Since my diagnosis, I have put strategies in place that I hoped would stop or at least slow the progression of both the PD and the cognitive impairment.

Exercise

All forms of exercise (aerobic, strength, and flexibility) have been proven to have beneficial effects for PWPs. There is evidence that exercise may slow progression of PD and reduce its symptoms. Sustained exertion that creates an elevated heart rate is recommended. Discuss with your doctor what type of exercise would be best for you.

With regard to Lewy body dementia, it is believed that a healthy lifestyle with a focus on exercise, mental stimulation, and nutrition may delay age-related dementia.[59] However, it does not appear that there is any strategy that will slow or stop the progression of Lewy body dementia once it has started.[60] In my case, I choose to err on the side of optimism and exercise regularly at our community recreation centers. I also enjoy biking, which I am able to do fairly aggressively (strenuous rides of 20 miles or more) and walking/hiking for an hour or more. I also participate at a less strenuous level in golf, tennis, snow skiing, and swimming.

Medication

I take six 25/100 mg levodopa/carbidopa (Sinemet) at approximately four-hour intervals and two 5 mg selegiline (morning and afternoon) for PD. I take an antidepressant, bupropion SR/150 mg (Wellbutrin) twice a day to help keep my mood positive and ward off depression that can lead to apathy. I do this because I recognize that chemical changes occurring in the brain with PD can cause depression. As I have already mentioned, I am using the Exelon patch (9.5 mg/one a day) and Namenda (10 mg/2 per day) for cognitive symptom relief. Dr. Kluger has told me that it is currently thought that PWPs respond well in some cases to the combination of these two medications.

That has certainly been the case with me. I also take lisinopril for blood pressure and simvastatin for cholesterol control.

Supplements

There are diverse opinions about the value of dietary supplements in general. The ones that Dr. Kluger and I, with support from UCH's Integrative Medicine team, have agreed on (all of which are thought by some to benefit cognition) are:

- Vitamin D/4000 IU (morning)
- Vitamin B12/1000 mg (morning)
- COQ10/800 mg (400 morning, 400 night)
- Acetyl L-carnitine/2 grams (1 morning, 1 night)

Other supplements and nonprescription medications that I take, which are unrelated (as far as I know) to cognition, are:

- Vitamin C/1000 mg (morning)
- Calcium magnesium w/D 1000/500/400 mg (2 in the morning, 1 at night) for bone strength
- Aspirin/81 mg (1 per day/pm), for cardiovascular precaution (family history of heart problems)
- Ibuprofen/200 mg (4 per day), for stiffness
- Prunelax (for constipation)

I believe that these are good choices based on the information available. I have recently learned that ibuprofen is being researched as a possible neuroprotective strategy (it may slow PD progression), as are caffeine and nicotine. Once again, share any ideas you would like to explore regarding medications, supplements, or exercise with your doctor. Patient engagement in these kinds of decisions should be viewed as positive by your doctor. If he or she is not open to your participation, consider changing doctors. I think it is accurate to say that Dr. Kluger and I think of our relationship as a partnership where both parties' input has value.

My PD symptoms remain generally mild. The fact remains that I have progressed to aMCI. According to Dr. Kluger, it is estimated that approximately 10-15% of those with aMCI progress to dementia annually. The bottom line is that although there is a significant chance that I will progress to dementia in the foreseeable future, it is not a foregone conclusion. I have not lost hope, and I don't want anyone in my position reading this book to lose hope either.

I received the following in an update from Johns Hopkins: "Staying mentally active by engaging in activities that challenge and stimulate the mind may be a key factor in maintaining memory and other cognitive skills, according to research from the *New England Journal of Medicine* and the Mayo Clinic."[61] In particular, I plan to stay engaged in activities about which I am passionate as long as possible. I believe that staying connected in this way is important.

For example, during July 2012 I sang in a patriotic fundraiser concert related to the Waldo Canyon fire in Colorado Springs being planned by the Tri-Lakes Music Association (a community organization dedication to promotion of the arts in the Monument, Colorado area). I was inspired to suggest to my community chorus that we could "recreate" this concert for our annual Veteran's Day program by singing to DVD accompaniment, using materials I was able to borrow (without violating copyright laws). They agreed, but it turned out that the only way this had a chance to work was if I would conduct (something I have never done, though I have many years of choral experience). In hindsight, I don't know what I was thinking when I took this on. Somewhere around mid-September I was starting to feel overwhelmed and knew that our chorus members might not understand my need to plan everything down to the letter and the mistakes I was making due to slowness and memory problems. I decided to come clean with them and shared the fact that I was having particular types of cognitive problems. From that point on it was clear, though nothing was said, that I had their compassion and support. This redoubled my dedication to seeing this program through in spite of the difficulties. The outcome and reaction from both the chorus and the community made it all worthwhile.

In the process, I learned that I was still able to do some things, even though it was hard, that I would have thought beforehand exceeded my current capabilities. I also learned that it sometimes helps to share your problems with others. As a result, I plan to intentionally set the bar a little higher than I might have before and share what I am experiencing more openly.

I hope that my clinical research activities will contribute to our understanding of PD and related problems, including cognition and memory impairments. In my younger years, I was not interested in organ donation. That has changed in recent years based on my commitment to the importance of research. I have made arrangements to donate my brain (and most of the rest of my body) to a facility in Los Angeles for research purposes. Unlike many other similar organizations, there is no cost associated with doing this. Since I planned to be cremated, why not make the ultimate contribution to research? For anyone who is interested, here is the contact information for this organization:

Human Brain & Spinal Fluid Resource Center

VA Greater Los Angeles Healthcare System

West Los Angeles Healthcare Center (127A)

11301 Wilshire Blvd

Los Angeles, CA 90073

(310) 268-3536 - Bank Office

(310) 268-4768 – FAX

Email: brainbnk@ucla.edu

Chapter 12: Impact on Families

Lewy body dementia is clearly very challenging, both for those afflicted and for their families. Losing a loved one to Lewy body dementia or Parkinson's disease dementia (very closely related) has got to be excruciating on many levels. It is not something that many of us would care to know about, not because we are "unfeeling," but for reasons similar to why we would not put our hand on a hot stove: We know it will be painful. However, there are situations where we need to know what to expect. I include a description of the seven stages of dementia in appendix B at the back of the book (these are general and apply to most forms of dementia, such as Alzheimer's, LBD, and PDD).

I am going to share three stories about families that are dealing with (or have dealt with in the past) Lewy body dementia (LBD) at different stages, which I hope will be useful in helping us better understand the real-life impact of this disease. The first is the story of an individual who has been diagnosed. The last two are recollections regarding loved ones who have died with LBD.

Post-Diagnosis Stage: Mary's Story

Linda and I have been very good friends with a couple we have known for 30 years. They are both in their late seventies, I think. I will refer to them as Mary and Bill to protect their privacy. We were visiting with them early in 2011 when Mary told us about being frustrated with health problems she had been experiencing. Without going into detail, her symptoms sounded very much to us like Parkinson's. She had an appointment shortly after we left with one of the top movement disorder neurologists in the country, who was able to confirm that she had PD. Whether or not he suspected there might be more to it than that, we don't know.

While a PD diagnosis is never good news, Mary was relieved to finally know what was wrong and to have such a good doctor to work with. Mary and Bill had been spending at least a few months each winter in a warm climate and returned to their home on the East Coast in May. During the summer of 2012, she met with another top movement disorder neurologist close to where they live "back East." This time she came home with a related but different diagnosis: Lewy body dementia (LBD).

We knew that Mary had been troubled for quite a few years by what she called "night terrors." This diagnosis caught me very much by surprise, in spite of the fact that I know a great deal about LBD. It wasn't clear how much Mary and Bill understood about what to expect. Fortunately, Linda and I have also met their children over the years, including a daughter (whom I will call Janet) who lives close to her parents on the East Coast and helps Mary and Bill in many ways. I was able to email her a few web addresses that quickly brought her up to speed.

There is a rather unique connection between Mary and me because of our shared health issues. Janet understands and appreciates the level of concern Linda and I both feel. She provides periodic updates on her mom's condition and how this is affecting her dad. I have met very few men who are as dedicated to taking care of their wives as Bill. They celebrated their 50th wedding anniversary, with their children in attendance, at least four years ago. They are continuing to enjoy life, their families, and each other as Mary's condition evolves, though I know that the uncertainty is challenging for them both.

Loss of a Family Member: Grace's Story

I met with a friend (whom I will call Grace) who lost her mother (here called Liz) to Lewy body dementia and agreed to share her story. I will use Frank for her dad's name. Again, I am using fictitious names to protect the family's privacy.

Grace was the youngest child of Liz and Frank. She grew up in the Northeast and had two older sisters who were 16 and 12 when Grace was born and a brother who was 14. Tragically, her brother had heart surgery before she was born and died from an air embolism during a second heart surgery after she was born.

Frank retired from his position as a corporate marketing executive with a well-known company after 35 years. Liz had been a musician and music teacher and also capably filled the role of wife to a high-level businessman. After retirement, Liz and Frank found an independent retirement community in the Orlando area, where they rented initially, and ended up living there for seven to eight years. While there, they enjoyed being involved members of the First Presbyterian Church, a reflection of the role that faith played in their lives. Grace, her sisters, and their boys visited Liz and Frank often during those years, taking advantage of the many activities available in that area.

After a few years, Frank found a new "prototype" continuous care retirement community (CCRC) in the Gainesville, Florida, area. He liked the fact that it offered a full range of living and care services, including totally independent patio homes, independent apartments, assisted living, and skilled nursing. He broke the news to his children on the occasion of his and Liz's 50th wedding anniversary. Though Grace's and her sisters' initial reaction was that it was "too soon" to move into a community that offered advanced health services, they realized that their dad had done his homework and that this move, which would take place in two years, was part of his commitment that neither he nor Liz would be a burden to his family in the future. It would not take long for all of them to realize that it was the perfect choice.

The new community exceeded Liz's and Frank's expectations, which were already high. They were impressed by the affiliation the community had with the University of Florida and its medical school. Medical school students worked there in various roles and several retired high-level administrators, including a former president of the university and his family, were charter member residents. As a result, Frank and Liz had access to a superior level of medical care.

It should be noted that Liz and Frank had been in an extremely serious car accident during February 1992 (shortly after Grace was married), when Frank was 65 and Liz was 62. Liz suffered a significant brain injury and both sustained neck fractures that required them to wear supportive halos. While there were no immediate signs of cognitive problems, this could well have been a causative factor related to the symptoms Liz developed later.

Within a couple of years, in 2001, when Liz was 72, she was diagnosed with "early onset dementia." This was not a complete surprise, as Liz and Frank had both noticed that she was having trouble balancing the checkbook, keeping track of what each light switch was for, and finding her way back from the local grocery store. She gradually stopped driving and cooking (meals were provided to residents). Within about a year, they knew Liz's illness was progressing and the term "Lewy body dementia" began to come up in doctor appointments. Frank continued to be her sole caregiver, but that became difficult when Liz started to experience falls and often got lost in their building.

Together with their medical team, Liz and Frank made the difficult decision to move Liz into skilled nursing (bypassing the typical intermediate move to assisted living). She lived in a private apartment in the same building as Frank for about a year. They both knew it was the right thing to do, but they were understandably sad.

The decision was made easier by problems Liz experienced following a second mastectomy due to a recurrence of an earlier bout of breast cancer. Liz was under general anesthesia for the surgery and the family felt that she was never the same after that. They estimated that she only regained 70-80% of her former lucidity following that surgery. After that, Frank decided to forgo any further MRIs or heroic measures, especially given the apparent impact of anesthesia.

After her move to skilled nursing, Liz began to experience increasing confusion. Frank visited her three times a day and tried bringing her back to their apartment a couple times, but realized that this only added to Liz's confusion. She was diagnosed with Lewy body dementia around this time. Liz had started to experience "Parkinsonian" symptoms, including slowed gait that forced her to use a walker. Another piece of the puzzle was that she had been experiencing REM sleep disorder (acting out dreams) since before moving to Gainesville. She had been taking Aricept earlier and now switched to Namenda, a drug prescribed for moderate to severe LBD.

After talking to the doctors and doing some research on their own, Grace and her sisters realized it was time to make every minute count. They began to visit frequently, accompanied by their husbands and children, so that they could have quality time together before Liz's condition deteriorated to the point where her issues would scare the kids.

Grace commented that her mom's nursing team and other staff members became "like members of the family" and that they clearly were "called" to do the work they were doing. Monthly "team" meeting were attended by Frank, members of Liz's medical team, social workers, and physical therapists to discuss Liz's status and decide on next steps. Less than a year after Liz moved to skilled nursing, the local hospice organization contacted Frank and recommended that Liz start receiving hospice care immediately. Liz was at increased risk for falls and had taken a bad one that was possibly caused by a stroke. Frank was reluctant to take that step, but agreed three months later.

So, after only a year in skilled nursing care, Liz transitioned to hospice care. By this time, Frank had made sure that her affairs were in order, including necessary legal documents that made her wishes clear. Liz became totally bedridden and incontinent. Her lucidity waned and, toward the end, Grace could only guess as to whether her mom knew who she was based on her facial expression. Frank, Grace, and her sisters made sure that Liz always had family with her. She died on Palm Sunday, 2010, nine years after being diagnosed with dementia, from complications related to LBD.

The family was obviously distraught, but was thankful that they had had time to say their goodbyes and that they had their faith, family, and friends to support them. They were extremely appreciative of the care Liz received from her medical team, especially hospice. Hospice did a great job of keeping them informed regarding what to expect, which was very important.

I asked Grace if she had any advice to offer families dealing with LBD. She said she would recommend taking advantage of hospice "sooner rather than later" and advised spending time with your loved one "early and often."

Frank is now 87 and showing the wear and tear that comes with age, as well as the stress of losing a child and his wife, a major car accident, and 35 years in a demanding job. He had a heart valve replacement about a year ago. Grace's brother-in-law is a CPA and is helping Frank by paying the bills; he will facilitate the type of problem-free transition that Frank desires for his family when the time comes for him to join Liz.

Loss of a Family Member: Kate's Story

This third account was written by Kate Kelsall, a personal friend and also a PWP, who writes an award-winning blog called "Shake, Rattle, and Roll." Kate lost her mom, aged 83, to Lewy body dementia in 2008 after more than three years of watching her deteriorate. These are excerpts from Kate's eloquent (and often humorous) account of this experience, which can be read in its entirety at http://katekelsall.typepad.com/my_weblog/lewy_body_dementia/:

> On an autumn day on October 6, 2005, our Irish clan piled in the office of Dr. Peter Holt, a geriatric internist in Kansas City. We were at the appointment to find out what ailed our 80-year-old Mom, Marge Doyle. When Dr. Holt opened the door to his office, he seemed surprised to see the Doyle family filling every inch of his

office space. He affectionately gave us the nickname of the Doylies.

Dr. Holt wheeled over to Mom in his chair so that he could talk to her face to face. He tried to get Mom to explain why she had this appointment today. Mom thought the Doylies had forced her to come.

Dr. Holt was concerned when he discovered that Mom had no medical records, although she lived in the Kansas City area her entire life. It's true – Mom never went to doctors except for the birth of her five children, with her youngest child being in her early forties. So we were starting from scratch here with no medical records.

My brother wrote a short history of Mom's medical problems from his memory and from photos of Mom to illustrate his points. One photo of Mom from a year earlier showed Mom appearing to weigh more than 200 pounds with her short 5'2" frame, while at today's appointment she weighed in at 98 pounds and looked like a malnourished concentration camp survivor. She hadn't even been on a diet, and no one could explain the weight loss.

Mom's problems seemed to have started with the turkey incident several years ago when she dropped her baked turkey on the kitchen floor on Thanksgiving morning. The turkey meltdown forced my brother to scrounge around Kansas City to locate a baked turkey for Thanksgiving dinner in a few hours.

My siblings discussed Mom's hallucinations (or as one of my sister called "Mom's little delusions"). Mom was preoccupied with death and destruction, killing all of us off in her mind, a new funeral everyday for her sisters, her kids and her grandkids. And her hallucinations were scary and terrifying.

"What are you doing here?" Mom asked my brother, "You're supposed to be dead. You can't keep coming back from heaven like this." For that moment my brother was the favored one, while the rest of us suffered in eternal damnation.

When Dr. Holt asked Mom her name, address and phone, she responded, "My name is Marjorie Doyle, and I live at 9235 Woodman. I know my name!" But she couldn't remember her phone number. She dismissed it with a chuckle saying "I never have to call myself." Now she can't remember any of these important demographics.

At that appointment, Mom started calling herself Miss Marjorie or Miss Margie, as though she's talking about another person. Marge and Mom were no longer in her vocabulary.

When the doctor asked Mom what day it was, I glanced at my daily calendar, so I could answer correctly. Mom didn't have a daily planner and didn't know the answer. And Mom's personality had recently changed. Her sweet, prim and proper, shy temperament had been replaced by cantankerous behavior and foul-mouthed language.

I was concerned that Mom might have Parkinson's disease. I told the doctor that I was diagnosed with Parkinson's ten years earlier, and that I observed Mom's stiffness and slowness when she moved, balance problems with always being on the verge of falling, her lack of facial expression, stooped shoulders and posture, and shuffling steps.

I gasped when Dr. Holt tested her balance by having Mom get up from the chair without using her hands. Mom nearly fell backwards.

At the conclusion of the appointment, Dr. Holt referred Mom to a neurologist. The neurologist confirmed Dr. Holt's suspicions of the diagnosis of Lewy Body Dementia (LBD), a disease that we never knew existed. LBD is the second most common kind of dementia, with Alzheimer's being the most common.

LBD is a complex blend of the confusion and memory loss of Alzheimer's Disease, the stiffness and slowness of Parkinson's Disease, and the hallucinations and delusions of Schizophrenia.

Symptomatically, this disease lies at the intersection of Alzheimer's and Parkinson's disease and was first fully recognized in 1996. The hallmark of Lewy body disease is the real clincher in this diagnosis: vivid and detailed hallucinations featuring friends and relatives. These phantasms are distressing, often terrifying. Finally, in Lewy body dementia, hallucinations occur early in the disease, frequently before the cognitive deficits are apparent.

It was a bittersweet experience when visiting Mom in Kansas City. I didn't know if Mom recognized me or what she was feeling or thinking. I tried to put myself in her position, and if she could communicate, this is what I imagined her saying.

- I used to be the Mom of this family. LBD is in charge of my body and mind and has turned me into an infant. Now I'm the baby of the family.

- My daughter, Pat, spoon-feeds me what suspiciously looks like baby food, sweet potatoes whirled in a blender.

- My son, Tom, bundles me in a blanket and walks me around the neighborhood in a wheelchair that looks like a stroller.

- My daughter, Denise, spreads my youthful Irish face with lotion and applies lipstick.

- My daughter, Kate from Denver, repeatedly says in a loud voice, "Mom, this is Kate, your oldest daughter." I am not deaf, but everyone talks to me as though I am.

- The "hired help" change my diapers and bathe me.

- My words come out like baby talk as they struggle to understand. It is easier to remain quiet, but sometimes I articulate a five-word lucid sentence, and everyone is surprised.

- "They came out real cute," I utter when shown a photo of my grandchildren.

- "We need a professional here," when my daughter, who is not a beautician, attempts to cut my hair.

- All my kids try to get a laugh or a smile out of me, their former Mom. I'm no longer the Mom but the baby of the family. I must now rely on them to mother me.

We fear that our Mom will either choke to death or starve to death.

Over the last three years she has been hospitalized a couple of times, but primarily she's remained in her own home with round the clock home health care.

Mom is now in a nursing home and has eaten and drunk very little in the past two weeks. When she is fed or provided liquid, she frequently chokes. Mom has the swallowing problems (dysphagia) so typical of Parkinson's patients. Aspiration pneumonia, a leading cause of death with Parkinson's patients, often develops as a complication of mealtime swallowing problems, leading to the inhalation of food and drink.

Approaching the end of her life, Mom has experienced a decrease in appetite and thirst, and wants little or no food or fluid. It's her body's way of preparing for the final shutdown: death. It's a predicament – death by choking or by death by starvation. My brothers, sisters and I have difficulty accepting that there's nothing more we can do, and that it's beyond our control.

Last week was a blur of events and emotions. Mom passed away Monday, October 27, 2008, with her five children, two sisters and one niece surrounding her. Although we have yet to see the death certificate, most likely the causes of death will be complications from Lewy Body Dementia (LBD) including dysphagia (difficulty swallowing) and malnutrition.

My family got Hospice involved on Friday, October 24 after Mom failed a swallowing test the previous day. She suffered from LBD for more than three years. Mom had eaten or drunk very little for nearly two weeks. My family declined a feeding tube knowing that Mom would not have wanted to continue suffering. On Friday, Hospice estimated that Mom had between two and seventy-two hours to live. Mom outlived their prediction by three hours.

By the time I arrived in Kansas City early Saturday morning, I was surprised that my siblings and aunts had come to terms with the inevitability of Mom's death. When I inquired about their change in attitude, they attributed it to the Hospice care team, particularly the volunteers, most of which had suffered similar losses, and were grateful for their assistance.

I never realized that the task of dying was so complicated. The body completes its natural process of shutting down. Throughout the final stages, Mom's respiration was measured and blood pressure, temperature, and pulse recorded. Mom's comfort was maximized and pain minimized through Morphine and Ativan administered orally by drops under her tongue. Her breathing pattern was irregular with either big intervals between each breath when she seemed to be not breathing or rapid shallow pant-like breathing. Mom's hands and arms seemed cool to the touch. The color on her feet and legs turned to purple as the circulation of her blood was decreasing. She seemed to be constantly sleeping and couldn't be aroused.

Mom deteriorated further on Monday. She nearly missed hearing farewells from two of her relatives. However, late morning, one of her daughter-in-laws stopped by to say her final goodbye.

Before she passed, my brother and I saw one tear falling from her right eye. Her breathing and heartbeat stopped at 3:36 PM, and she died peacefully. I was honored to be part of the dying process. Through Hospice, Mom died with dignity and respect.

I can't read these accounts without feeling the anguish these families have gone through. At the same time, I recognize the opportunity we all have to provide our loved ones and plan for ourselves an "exit strategy" that promotes peace, closure, and (if one so chooses) hope for what lies beyond death.

Chapter 13: Palliative Care and Neurology: Striving for Justice

The following are excerpts from an email that I sent to Dr. Kluger in May 2013:

> I have been thinking about our conversation on Monday regarding the desirability of doctors having a more personal understanding of patients. Even if a doctor sees the potential benefits (which I do not think they all do), this would require a high level of commitment in a world where disposable time is a precious commodity. I can understand that some are reluctant to break through the "protective space" between them and patients. By doing this, they risk losing some degree of their clinical objectivity that some would argue is necessary to provide optimum care. I, and Dr. Graboys (and you, I think) would

argue the opposite. How can a doctor hope to provide "optimum care" if they look no further than what is written on charts and records and reflected in tests? Yes, there is risk involved. Including the risk of having an emotional stake in the lives (and deaths) of their patients. And yet, isn't that what being a doctor is supposed to be about? Making a difference in the quality of the lives of patients? Is it really possible to do one without the other? It seems that the Hippocratic Oath supports this concept:

"That above all else I will serve the highest interests of my patients through the practice of my science and my art"

Taking it a step further, this goes on to state:

"That I will be an advocate for patients in need and strive for justice in the care of the sick."

How can a doctor advocate properly for a patient, let alone "strive for justice," if they do not "know" them? This "striving for justice" is, in my opinion, central to the issue of what palliative care should be all about.

A note of explanation is required here. My comments to Dr. Kluger involved a subject I have thought about a great deal and about which I have strong feelings, which probably explains the outspoken tone. I have nostalgic "Welby-esque" (people under 50 will likely have no idea what I am talking about—this refers to a TV show, *Marcus Welby MD*,[62] about a family doctor from the 1960s) memories of trips to the doctor in my youth when doctors knew their patients on a personal level. Over the years, as these visits have evolved from patient-centered care to what I call "industrialized medicine,"[63] where doctors are increasingly specialized, work in teams, and rarely have the time or inclination to "know" their patients, I have experienced a sense of loss and even betrayal. It has been an insidious change (and not all bad) that should have been predictable based on the amount of time that doctors have to spend on the paperwork that, along with serving a useful purpose, must be done to satisfy the requirements of insurance companies and protect themselves from lawsuits.

When I think about patient-centered care, I am reminded of my former life in the retail and direct marketing business world. It became second nature for me to approach problems using a framework that included strategic planning[64] and management by objectives (MBO).[65] I learned the importance of being goal-directed. As more sophisticated technology was developed, marketing evolved from a "shotgun" approach, using a mix of media in an attempt to maximize business with a broad audience, to "targeted marketing,"[66] where we began to understand the importance of knowing who our customer was and designing promotions that would appeal to that particular customer. The next step was the era of total quality management (TQM),[67] in which businesses began to recognize that they could maximize customer loyalty by understanding more about the needs and wants of customer segments and devising strategies to consistently meet or exceed their expectations. Today, this approach has been further refined with customer relationship management (CRM),[68] which uses advanced technologies (such as "cloud-based" sales and marketing information systems) to provide detailed, ongoing insights regarding target customers. Which leads me (finally) to my point: To succeed in today's highly competitive global environment where customers have more choices than ever, businesses *must* be "customer-centric,"[69] because having the *right* goals is absolutely critical.

In short, the business world has learned the importance of understanding who the customer is, communicating with customers on an ongoing basis to understand what is important to them, and developing strategic plans designed to consistently meet or exceed their expectations. It seems to me that the same principles apply (or should apply) to patient-centered care: The customer is the patient and, secondarily, the patient's family (not the hospital or insurance companies). I am not trying to be condescending or preachy, but I feel that I owe it to my fellow patients to be clear about this. There must be two-way communication with patients to understand their needs and wants, and this must be factored into a plan for delivery of outstanding medical care using the best available knowledge and technology. As a result, this plan should include a commitment to patient empathy and engagement. Finally, the plan should be designed to allow providers to obtain feedback from patients that will enable them to determine the degree to which they are meeting their own goals.

Some may say I am dreaming. But like John Lennon wrote in "Imagine," I'm not the only one. I'm not saying this will be easy, or that it can be achieved overnight. I am particularly worried right now as we stand on the brink of instituting socialized medicine[70] in the United States. The preceding endnote provides a list of pros and cons on this subject, which will enable you to reach your own conclusion about whether this is good or bad.

I know that some hospitals and doctors are already utilizing at least some of the strategies I have recommended. For example, my hospital (University of Colorado Hospital) emails a short survey to me following each visit to get feedback on their performance and my level of satisfaction. I am particularly encouraged by a program for neurological palliative care that Dr. Kluger started at UCH in March 2013 (before he had the benefit of my "wisdom" as expressed in the email I sent him in May). To me this shows that our thoughts have been evolving in similar directions on parallel paths and that we have reached a confluence precipitated by his involvement with this book.

At the beginning of September 2013, Benzi (we are now on a first-name basis) enlisted me to help publicize a presentation he was planning, titled "Palliative Care and Neurology: Time for a Paradigm Shift." He knew that I was disappointed at being unable to attend, so he invited me to an Epilepsy and Movement Disorders symposium he hosted on September 21, 2013, that included his palliative care presentation. I was extremely energized and encouraged by what he had to say to his fellow neurology professionals. Since then, I have learned that he is working with a Canadian colleague, Dr. Janis Miyasaki, on development of this new model. Elements of interest to me include:

- The need for palliative care for PD patients begins at diagnosis. Currently, they are typically given minimal information and then set adrift until their next appointment (typically in about three months). This is a time when the patient and family often need to ask questions and process predictable emotions.

- The need for palliative care continues to grow from the time of diagnosis, and at some point may transition to a focus on hospice (part of the palliative care spectrum, but not the same thing). The primary goal of palliative care is prevention and relief of suffering for patients and their families, including control of pain and other physical symptoms as well as psychological, social, and spiritual issues. It affirms and supports life while addressing death as a normal and expected outcome.

- Palliative care can be used alone or in conjunction with curative treatments and requires a team approach (neurologist, internist, psychologist, social worker, hospice, clergy, etc.).

- Hospice is the last stage in a palliative care spectrum that includes end-of-life care for the patient and family and a focus on comfort and quality of life.

- Caregiver needs must be addressed, including burnout, spiritual needs, and demoralization.
- Most neurologists receive little or no palliative care training.
- Many doctors are reluctant to discuss difficult subjects like cognitive issues or death with patients.
- Communication with patients and families is a core issue. Good communication includes adequate time for questions, clear explanation of the meaning of a diagnosis, provision of information on where to go for support, and appropriate delivery of bad news.

Patients need to view palliative care as a two-way street and learn what they need to do to fulfill their role in the process. There are a variety of steps available to take in preparation for death that enable us to manage this transition and minimize problems for our loved ones, including wills, living wills, powers of attorney, advance directives regarding health care, establishment of trusts, and more.[71] Our church had a presentation on a type of planning that involves creation of a document called "Five Wishes," which communicates information to a trusted individual. The "Wishes" document could include preferences regarding burial, donation of body parts, and memorial/funeral services; disposition of valued personal items; elimination of online accounts and footprints, handling of computer files, and lists of user names and passwords; and any other specific desires or guidance regarding end-of-life wishes. Of course, we have the option to let someone else worry about these details, because we prefer not to think about them, but this does not seem fair or considerate to me. I chose to share a "last wishes" document with my older son, along with the comment that I hoped it would not be needed for many years.

Families need to be as knowledgeable as possible regarding their loved one's illness so they can advocate for them appropriately to (and even after) the end. As much as we would like to rely on doctors and nurses to know everything they need to know to provide optimum care, that is not always possible; in addition, often they do not have the legal authority to do what "ought" to be done. For example, families need to be aware that most patients enter hospice too late or not at all. When asked, after their loved one has passed, what they would do differently, many families say that they would have engaged hospice sooner. Talk to your doctor about how to know when the time is right. Understand that, even though it is difficult, the time will come when it is no longer appropriate to try to prolong life. At that point, the objective should shift to meeting the patient's emotional and spiritual needs as death approaches. This is the time when advance directives become crucial in allowing the patient to die according to his or her wishes. This is obviously in the best interests of the patient and also benefits the family by facilitating closure and a sense of peace.

The questions surrounding a patient's wishes about how he or she wants to die and his or her right to choose are controversial due to cultural, religious, and legal constraints. It seems to me that we are at a point where it is appropriate for reasonable people to re-examine some of our long-standing positions about moral and legal restrictions placed on the options that people with terminal illnesses (including dementia) can choose from when making end-of-life choices and decisions. Dementia poses a serious problem—on the verge of being an epidemic in this nation—the financial and emotional costs of which are significant. If individuals face the possibility of eventually being unable to communicate with or even recognize those they love most, with no reasonable hope of recovery, should they not have the option of developing a plan to end their own lives? Should they be forced to suffer needlessly while their families watch helplessly?

I urge patients and families to plan a meeting with their doctor and other hospice team members to discuss this subject openly, to help the patient reach a decision that is appropriate for him or her and develop consensus with family members. This should include a frank discussion about how a "natural death" is likely to occur. Topics the doctor could be asked to explain include euthanasia (not legal in the United States, but currently available in the Netherlands, Belgium, and Luxembourg), physician-assisted suicide (legal currently in the states of Oregon, Vermont, Washington, and Montana), and terminal sedation. Also discuss the pros and cons of aggressive symptom treatment and life-prolonging strategies. Once the patient reaches a decision, his or her wishes should be legally documented in writing to avoid any future complications or confusion.

Regarding the spiritual component of palliative care, UCH studies indicate that spiritual and well-being support services are associated with higher patient quality of life. More than 70% of PD patients reported that spirituality/faith was important to their lives, and more than 50% use prayer to help with their health concerns.

Learning about Benzi's plans for palliative care at my hospital and his thoughts about the need to understand and honor patient end-of-life choices has given me a tremendous sense of peace about the process of dying. It was the piece that had been missing. The other piece—already in place—is my faith.

Chapter 14: Faith

I have always been interested in TV programs like Carl Sagan's "Cosmos" and books that discuss the nature of the universe. I recently read a few chapters of *A Brief History of Time* by Stephen Hawking, which include an explanation of quantum mechanics/physics (the two terms seem to be used interchangeably). I started piecing together a hypothesis related to the subatomic particles (quarks) that everything is made of, including the human body. I think it is accurate to refer to these as "energy particles." I also have read *Proof of Heaven* by Dr. Eban Alexander, in which he describes his extended near-death experience (NDE) in vivid detail. He speaks of being in the presence of an entity that he knew was God. His description is mesmerizing, but he is clear about the fact that any words he has would not do justice to this entity, which he calls "Om."

Another thought that has occurred to me is that the way we (as humans) tend to think of God probably confuses things. However, it is understandable that we would create an image that we can wrap our minds around. This is reminiscent of the movie *Contact* (based on the book by Carl Sagan), in which an astronomer turned astronaut travels through a "wormhole" to a distant part of the universe and finds herself on what appears to be a familiar beach in Florida, conversing with an unidentified entity that has taken the form of her father to facilitate communication.

In time, I synthesized these concepts and came to see that a legitimate case could be made for the possibility that, when we die, our "energy" somehow returns to the universe that is Om's domain. I am probably going to lose some credibility here (not that I ever had much to begin with), but the concept of "The Force" from *Star Wars* comes to mind, along with the concept that the "Om entity" controls it and everything else in the universe (or universes).

I suggest that what may happen to our "energy" once it is returned to the universe is in God's hands, as is everything else. By the way, I don't see this theory as contradicting the existence of Jesus for Christians. I don't know enough about other religions to comment on how these ideas might be in accord with or conflict with the tenets of Buddhism, Islam, Judaism, or Hinduism, for example, but my sense is that they would not be entirely incompatible. In any case, it is just a hypothesis.

I will admit that I am encouraged by this conjecture. It is not likely, or even important, in my opinion, that we will ever have all the answers to these timeless questions—not that I think it is a bad thing to seek them, which is human nature after all. What is most important to me is that I try to live my life in a way that will please God.

I am not angry at God, nor do I blame Him for my illness. I understand that He does not cause bad things to happen to people. I am truly able to consider the prospect of death without the trepidation I would have experienced when I was younger. The knowledge that God's love is unconditional, that His grace will continue to surround my family after I'm gone, and that "a room has been prepared for me" in His house, removes the fear (for both the present and the future) that I might otherwise feel.

I do not try to force my beliefs on anyone. I realize that not everyone agrees with me or shares my views. I will say that I wish everyone could experience the joy and relief of not having to be in charge and the knowledge that God will be waiting for all of us at the end of our journeys.

Chapter 15: Recommendations

I have had the privilege of speaking to many PD support groups and written numerous blog articles that have forced me to think about what I believe is of primary importance to PWPs and care partners for living with PD and maintaining a good quality of life. I hope that these recommendations, based on my experience and the feedback of others, are useful.

For PWPs:

1. **Be sure your doctor is a movement disorder specialist/neurologist (MDS/MDN).** Even if your doctor is a neurologist, this does not mean that he or she has the experience or education with movement disorders that will enable him or her to provide the specific care that you need.

Visit http://www.pdf.org/en/yy_doctor for a list of MDSs in your state. If your insurance company prevents you from seeing an MDS, let them know that this is a serious problem for you and seek a referral. If you cannot find or get access to one, let your local support group leaders know so they can report it to the regional PD organization for follow-up. If you have this type of insurance company problem, or if there are no MDSs located in your area, find a neurologist who has demonstrable experience in working with PD.

2.   **Exercise.** There are many things related to PD that are beyond your control. Getting regular exercise is something you *can* control that can make a big difference in your symptoms and your quality of life. Establish a plan with your MDS that is appropriate based on your age and condition. Try to choose exercise that you enjoy. Remember that physical and mental exercise are equally important!

3.   **Participate in clinical research trials.** When you do this, you accomplish two things. First, you help with the advancement of knowledge that will lead to a cure. Second, you learn things that may help you. Information

on specific studies, including availability, location, and timing of research trials, visit https://foxtrialfinder. michaeljfox.org/.

4.   **Learn everything you can about PD.** This applies to both PWPs and care partners. By doing this, you will have a better idea of what to expect in terms of symptoms and progression. Also, it will enable both of you to advocate for yourselves, ask informed questions, and become active/proactive in the management of your health. For a list of online information resources, visit http://shakypawsgrampa.blogspot.com/2011/12/ resource-list-donation-appeal.html. Also try Googling any combination of "Parkinson's" and "_____" (fill in the blank with any topic of interest, such as fatigue, non-motor symptoms, or cognition). Choose relatively current articles by recognizable organizations for the most reliable information.

5.   **Prepare for your MDS appointments.** Remember that MDSs are very busy individuals who want to provide you with the best care possible. Help make the limited time you have together in appointments productive by preparing a list that includes:

- Your current list of **prescriptions**, including dose size and times/day you take that dose.

- Your current list of **supplements**, including dose size and times/day you take that dose.

- List of **current symptoms** in order of how troublesome they are to you. Use bold type to identify the most troublesome symptoms.

- A list of **observations/information** regarding your condition or any changes that you want your MDS to know about. Record on/off fluctuations, episodes of dyskinesia, and whether they occur at the peak or end of the medication cycle.

- A list of **questions** regarding your condition, symptoms, treatment, medications, alternative therapies, or new developments you have heard about that may apply to you. It is extremely important that you and your care partner give this careful thought in advance. By organizing for your appointment this way, there should be adequate time to have all your questions answered. If your care partner is unavailable to attend the appointment, then choose a friend or relative to accompany you. It's important to have two sets of eyes and ears and someone to take notes.

6. **If you are not comfortable with your MDS for any reason, talk to him or her about it.** If you don't understand your treatment plan, can't get answers to your questions, can't obtain needed referrals, are unable to communicate with your MDS between appointments in a reasonable manner, or anything else, *talk about it.* Be a polite squeaky wheel. If you are unable to resolve problems that are important to you, find another MDS! Your number-one obligation is to yourself and your care partner.

7. **Attempt to "live in the moment" as much as possible.** Learn from the past and move on. Plan for the future, but do not dwell on the uncertainty that it surely contains. I know that this is easier said than done. In my case, I rely on my faith for reassurance and guidance.

8. **Set meaningful goals and work to accomplish them.** If this has always been your approach, continue it. If it has not, resolve to start. There is no shortage of opportunities, as we all know. Choose from things like reaching out to help others, treating your care partner with patience and

respect, maintaining wellness, getting exercise (physical and mental), writing a memoir, attending seminars, participating in clinical research studies, participating in PD fundraisers, attending support group meetings, attending church or otherwise engaging your faith, and many more. Make your goals as specific as possible and make sure you are prepared and able to do what is required to accomplish them. Hold yourself accountable and ask your care partner to do the same.

9.   **Stay in touch with your passions.** Some of the non-motor problems associated with PD can include depression, anxiety, and apathy. You may be able to reduce these kinds of issues by engaging in activities that have been important to you in the past. If they involve physical or mental challenges you are no longer up to, try modified versions or seek new activities related to your passion (such as listening to music or attending concerts if you are no longer able to sing or play an instrument). Resolve to stay engaged with family and friends. It is okay to give yourself permission to have a "down day" once in a while, but don't stay there.

10. **Continue to seek and live your "personal truth" without trying to force it on others.** I picked up this concept in a book titled *Wisdom of the Ages* by Wayne Dyer. That book speaks to the desirability of each individual taking ownership of what they choose to believe and let these choices, not the opinions or positions of others, guide how they live their lives.

For Care Partners:

1. **Live in the moment.**

   - Learn from the past and plan for tomorrow, but live for today. What do you believe in and what matters most to you? Do your actions reflect your beliefs and priorities? Talk about these things with your care partner and discuss any changes you might want to make as part of a plan for the future.

   - Don't put off those activities that you have talked about doing "some day."

   - Make time for fun.

2. **Communicate**

   - It is crucial to keep the lines of communication open. Tell each other what you are thinking and feeling.

- Share the things you are worried about and problem-solve together. Express your love for each other frequently.

- Catch each other doing little things that provide an opportunity to express appreciation.

3. **Learn**

- Learn as much as you can about PD and related issues.

- Stay engaged by participating in support groups and seminars.

- Participate in clinical research trials with your partner, in order to help yourselves as well as others.

- Understand and accept that PD is a moving target and that your partner's evolving condition/needs—as well as your own—will require flexibility and adaptation.

4. **Advocate for your partner and yourself**

- Accompany your partner to all medical appointments to get and provide first-hand information about what your partner is experiencing as well as being a second set of ears.

- Because it is typical for your partner to have executive function problems, take notes regarding important details.

- Ask questions, voice thoughts and ideas, and ask for clarification of anything that is unclear.

5. **Take care of yourself**

- Ask for help. Solicit assistance as needed from family members and/or friends.

- Make time for yourself. Stay engaged with your passions.

- Attend to your personal wellness.

6. **Faith**

- Our belief that we will be equipped to deal with whatever happens is extremely comforting to Linda and me. Staying committed to that idea over time requires faith.

- Faith provides an opportunity to let go of fear about the future over which we have no control, and focus on the things we can control.

7. **Patience**

- PD mood swings and/or cognitive problems can be very hard on relationships. No matter how good your communication, it is likely that your partner will sometimes act or react in ways that are not tactful or appropriate. Try very hard not to take these things personally.

- At a later time, communicate about what happened.
- Don't let an individual episode create a rift between you.
- Talk with your partner's MDS about any ongoing concerns.

8. Balance

- Your "PD life" takes place in the context of your overall life. It will be beneficial for both of you to keep the two integrated and balanced as much as possible.
- As the disease evolves, your partner's physical and mental abilities will change and may be influenced by depression, anxiety, or apathy.
- Based on your knowledge of your partner, you can experiment with different strategies to encourage exercise, keep him or her engaged mentally and socially, discourage driving, and more. Keep your MDS in the loop and ask for suggestions.

- Care partner/PWP breakout sessions in support group meetings are a good opportunity to share concerns and get suggestions.

9. **Be prepared to make tough choices**

- Despite your best efforts, there may be a time when you are no longer able to cope with your partner at home by yourself.

- Explore options (preferably with your partner) such as assisted living, residential facilities, or in-home care/services so that you can make an informed decision if and when the time comes.

- Do not suffer in silence or feel compelled to go down with the ship. Talk to your MDS, support group friends, and family members as necessary.

10. **Perspective**

- Continue to find the joy in your lives and the love in your relationship.

- Celebrate the small victories.

- Be happy whenever possible.

- Do NOT let PD own you!

Epilogue

Linda and I returned to Mt. Elbert in August 2013 with our close friends, Bill and JoAnn Schmitz, and were able to get the same campsite we had in 2007 at Elbert Creek Campground (one of the top-rated campgrounds in the United States). We have camped over the years at many beautiful places with Bill and JoAnn, but they had never been to this campground. After setting up their newly acquired pop-up camper around 8:00 p.m. on Friday night (they are both still working), we enjoyed the campfire with the sound of the rushing water as a backdrop. The next morning, after seeing the campsite in the light of day, including our private "alcove" on the shore of the stream, they told us that this was the best camping spot they had ever seen in Colorado.

We had talked about trying to hike all the way up to the top again, but this time we planned to park in the south parking lot and take the easier trail both ways. We had scoped out the parking area the day before our friends arrived and were ready to go. This time we would be properly prepared and have plenty of water.

In hindsight, I don't know what I was thinking. We had heard about a new movement disorder team in the Denver area, Dr. Monica Giroux and Sierra Ferris, and their exploits with leading groups of patients on climbs at places like Mt. Kilimanjaro in Kenya, so I suppose I thought doing Mt. Elbert (which I had already done before) should be realistic. Also, Linda and I had walked with our son and three of our grandchildren in the "Bolder Boulder" 10K fundraiser on Memorial Day. We had been getting plenty of exercise during the summer. What I failed to take into account was the fact that, although I completed it, I was a wreck after walking that 10K on level ground at around 6000 feet elevation.

Luckily, Bill (who has climbed quite a few "fourteeners") told me he wasn't planning to go to the top and would prefer to do some less aggressive hiking. I acquiesced, saying that we would do whatever they would like to do. So we headed up the Colorado Trail from our campsite at 10,000 feet elevation toward the north Mt. Elbert trailhead, which starts below the treeline at about 11,500 feet. The idea was to continue on the Colorado Trail rather than going up Mt. Elbert.

We set off at a fairly brisk (for me) pace. I was using my ski poles to help with balance and to propel myself up hills (I use rubber-tipped walking poles at home, which I highly recommend for PWPs). The trail became narrow and winding as we ascended. It didn't take long for me to feel the altitude, which increased my unsteadiness. The trail, which was carved into the side of the mountain, was steeply uphill on one side and downhill on the other, and I started to become apprehensive, especially when I had to stop to let someone go by. Nevertheless, I continued up the trail through many switchbacks until I realized I should turn around and go back down while Linda, JoAnn, and Bill went on. As it turned out, this was a good decision. My legs became increasingly rubbery and by the time I got to the bottom, I was doing the "PD shuffle" big time. No amount of adrenaline or commitment would have allowed me to make it up that mountain!

The writing of this book has been an important part of my journey. My initial attempts led to frustration over "false summits" similar to what we had experienced on our first Mt. Elbert climb. However, I persevered in spite of the fact that I had no clear idea about how I was going to reach my destination of finishing a book that "felt right." There were definitely peaks and valleys in the process. I realize now that I was trying to create something that felt "perfect," which was the wrong goal; my real hope has been to share something that will make a difference in people's lives.

I have often seen listings of programming on the Science Channel that I would have loved to watch. Unfortunately, that channel was not included in our cable TV package, and I was reluctant to upgrade due to the cost. Recently, I was surprised to find that I now have access to that channel. I have been like a pig in mud recording programs on the origins of the universe, our sun and the other stars, our solar system, our planet, and life on earth.

A big part of the joy of camping in Colorado for me has been the awesome panorama of the night sky at 10,000 feet. I am amazed every time I see it by the sheer number of stars, especially compared to the view at lower altitude in more densely populated areas. The Science Channel allows me to experience the views seen by those who seek to unravel the mysteries of deep space using technologies such as the Hubble telescope.

Just the other day I watched a program on the life cycle of stars[72] and the important role their deaths play for future life in our universe. When viewed from a distance, all the stars seem pretty much the same, and in fact they all do share certain characteristics,[73] but we now know that each star is unique based on size, composition, mass, heat, gravity, brightness, and more. Even so, all stars eventually collapse and implode, ejecting elements vital to future life into the universe. Depending on their mass, all stars continue to exist in new forms (black dwarfs, neutron stars, or black holes) after their death.[74] When they die, they generate blasts of light and energy that travel through space at the speed of light,[75] which can be seen for as many as millions of years depending on proximity.

I can't accept that the sudden opportunity to watch these programs as I searched for a way to finish this book was a coincidence. The life cycle of stars is, for me, an appealing metaphor for all our lives. We are born and live lives that generate light and energy in ways that at first glance appear to be very similar. However, there is an undeniable uniqueness that becomes evident upon closer examination. As Jimmy Stewart's character in *It's a Wonderful Life* discovers, we all have an impact on the world around us. I like to think that when my time on earth is over, hopefully many years from now, my light and energy will live on in a different form that still has meaning. It has been, after all, a life filled with treasures beyond hope.

TREASURES BEYOND HOPE

Childhood dreams of love realized so soon
Not fully appreciated or understood
A timeless, priceless gift from God
Rushing to achieve and obtain
Often unaware of the riches before me
Always searching. Not satisfied.
Spiritual awakening, a life's journey
Growing closer to the finish
I feel the brush of angels' wings
As God writes the final chapter
And find comfort in the knowledge
That He will never leave our sides.
He will prepare a room for those who love Him
And that is all I need to know.
I will be eternally grateful for His gift of
Treasures wondrous beyond hope.

Kirk W. Hall

Appendix A: Technical Information

Parkinson's Disease Dementia (PDD)[76]

PD is a common disorder of deep brain structures that help control movement. Over time, many people with Parkinson's Disease develop Parkinson's Disease Dementia. Even younger people with Parkinson's Disease can develop dementia—one community-based study found that just over one person in ten with Parkinson's Disease between the ages of 50 and 60 had already developed dementia.

In Parkinson's disease, an abnormal protein [**Protein:** A molecule that consists of amino acids linked together. They are responsible for regulating many of the processes of our body.] accumulates inside neurons in deep brain structures known as the *substantia nigra*. This abnormal accumulation of what is called "alpha-synuclein" was first described by a Professor Lewy and still bears the name of being a "Lewy body." [**Lewy bodies:** Round clumps of protein found in the brain's neurons in many people who experience a neurodegenerative disorder.] Lewy bodies are also seen outside the deep brain structures, in the "thinking" parts of the brain in Parkinson's Disease Dementia and in Lewy body dementia. . . .

In Parkinson's Disease, one of the chief abnormalities is loss of the brain chemical (neurotransmitter) [**Neurotransmitter:** A specialized chemical messenger such as acetylcholine, that sends a message from one nerve cell to another. Neurotransmitters are responsible for the communication within the brain and also between the brain and other parts of the body.] dopamine. [**Dopamine:** A neurotransmitter found in the brain that has been associated with Parkinson's disease.] The usual treatment consists of medications that can increase the levels of dopamine, either by supplying more of it, or by slowing its breakdown.

Lewy Body Dementia (LBD)[77]

LBD is not a rare disease. It affects an estimated 1.3 million individuals and their families in the United States. Because LBD symptoms can closely resemble other more commonly known diseases like Alzheimer's and Parkinson's, it is currently widely underdiagnosed. Many doctors or other medical professionals still are not familiar with LBD.

LBD is an umbrella term for two related diagnoses. LBD refers to both Parkinson's disease dementia and dementia with Lewy bodies. The earliest symptoms of these two diseases differ, but reflect the same underlying biological changes in the brain. Over time, people with both diagnoses will develop very similar cognitive, physical, sleep, and behavioral symptoms.

While it may take more than a year or two for enough symptoms to develop for a doctor to diagnose LBD, it is critical to pursue a formal diagnosis. Early diagnosis allows for important early treatment that may extend quality of life and independence.

LBD is a multisystem disease and typically requires a comprehensive treatment approach. This approach involves a team of physicians from different specialties who collaborate to provide optimum treatment of each symptom without worsening other LBD symptoms. Many people with LBD enjoy significant improvement of their symptoms with a comprehensive approach to treatment.

Diagnostic Criteria[78]

Lewy body dementias include two clinical diagnoses, dementia with Lewy bodies (DLB) and Parkinson's disease dementia (PDD), which share essentially the same array of symptoms.

DLB Diagnostic Criteria

The diagnostic criteria for **probable DLB** require:

- The presence of dementia
- At least two of three core features:
    - fluctuating attention and concentration,
    - recurrent well-formed visual hallucinations, and
    - spontaneous parkinsonian motor signs.

Suggestive clinical features include:

- Rapid eye movement (REM) sleep behavior disorder
- Severe neuroleptic sensitivity
- Low dopamine transporter uptake in basal ganglia demonstrated by SPECT or PET imaging

In the absence of two core features, the diagnosis of **probable DLB** *can also be made if dementia plus at least* **one suggestive feature** *is present* **with one core feature**.

Possible DLB *can be diagnosed with the presence of* **dementia plus one core or suggestive feature**.

Supportive clinical features include repeated falls, syncope, a transient loss of consciousness, severe autonomic dysfunction, depression, systematized delusions, or hallucinations in other sensory and perceptual modalities. While these features may support the clinical diagnosis, they lack diagnostic specificity and can be seen in other neurodegenerative disorders.

These criteria have a sensitivity of 83% (17% clinical false negative rate) and a specificity of 95% (clinical false positive rate of only 5%) for the presence of neocortical Lewy bodies (LBs) at autopsy, the current diagnostic gold standard. However, these criteria are more predictive of autopsied cases with the relatively rare "pure" form of LBD rather than the much more common cases with a mixture of LBD and the pathology of AD [Alzheimer's disease]. The criteria cannot reliably differentiate between the two clinical entities. The DLB criteria tangentially address PDD as very similar to DLB with the exception of temporal appearance of extrapyramidal signs (i.e., in PDD the motor symptoms precede the onset of dementia by at least one year).

The current absence of radiological or biological markers that can reliably aid in the diagnosis of DLB has led to a search for clinical measures that can serve as markers for pathology or predictors of disease progression. Moreover, there is also an absence of effective treatment for DLB, except for drugs that offer modest control of the cognitive and behavioral symptoms. There are as yet no therapies that have proven to alter or delay disease progression. Early clinical detection of dementia or the identification of pre-clinical markers of different dementia pathologies may provide insight into early disease mechanisms and pave the way for the development of disease modifying therapy, which of necessity must be initiated at the earliest possible juncture, ideally before symptoms have developed.

The importance of early, aggressive treatment is supported by recent data suggesting that LBD patients might have better responses to cholinesterase inhibitors than AD patients. In addition, an early diagnosis of LBD implies that treating physicians will know to avoid medications that can aggravate the clinical picture, such as the traditional neuroleptics. It is estimated that almost 60% of LBD patients may exhibit exaggerated extrapyramidal signs, sedation, immobility, or neuroleptic malignant syndrome (NMS) with fever, generalized rigidity and muscle breakdown following exposure to neuroleptics. NMS is a life-threatening condition and the higher prevalence in LBD suggests that traditional neuroleptics such as haloperidol, fluphenazine or thioridazine should be avoided.

Early diagnosis will also allow families and caregivers the time to plan for the expected decline. Preventive steps to improve safety in the home environment should be taken, given the tendency to recurrent falls and rapid attentional fluctuations. Families will also have time to develop a better understanding of their role in patient care, including assistance with daily activities and provision of social and cognitive stimulation.

PDD Diagnostic Criteria

A consensus statement by a task force from the Movement Disorder Society for the diagnosis of PDD has just been published, providing criteria for probable and possible PDD.

A diagnosis of probable PDD requires the core features (Table 1) and a typical presentation of clinical features which is defined as having deficits in at least two out of four cognitive domains (below). There may or may not be behavioral symptoms, although their presence would support a diagnosis of probable PDD. There must not be any features present from groups III and IV, as the abnormalities and conditions described in these categories can cause too much uncertainty in a potential diagnosis.

A diagnosis of possible PDD also requires the core features, but can have a more non-characteristic pattern of symptoms in at least one of the cognitive domains. There may or may not be any behavioral symptoms. One or more features of group III may be present, and none in Group IV.

Table 1. Features of dementia associated with Parkinson's disease

Group I—The core feature requires a prior diagnosis of Parkinson's disease, and dementia causing a decline in function severe enough to impair the patient in daily activities and in at least one cognitive domain.

Group II—The clinical features include both the cognitive and behavioral domains described below:

Cognitive domains:

- Attention—The patient shows a level of impairment in attention, which may fluctuate over time
- Executive function—Impairment in complex thought processes such as in initiating an action, planning, or organization

- Visuo-spatial ability—Marked deficits in the processing of visuospatial material

- Memory—There is noticeable impairment in both the recall of existing memories and in the learning of new material

- Language—Basic language features are largely intact, although there may be difficulties in finding words and understanding complex sentences.

Behavioral domains:

- Apathy—Decreased spontaneity, motivation, effortful behavior

- Changes in personality and mood—Can include depression and anxiety

- Hallucinations—Usually complex and visual

- Delusions—Usually paranoid delusions, such as infidelity or perceived unknown guests in the home

- Excessive daytime sleepiness

Group III—The third category includes two features that will not rule out a diagnosis of PDD, but may make the diagnosis more uncertain:

- Existence of an abnormality such as vascular disease which causes cognitive impairment although not determined to cause dementia

- If the duration of time between the onset of motor and cognitive symptoms is not known

Group IV—The last domain contains two features which suggest that other existing conditions impair the patient's cognitive functioning to such an extent that reliable diagnosis of PDD becomes impossible.

- Cognitive or behavioral symptoms which occur only in the context of existing conditions, such as systemic diseases, drug intoxication, or major depression

- Symptoms compatible with vascular dementia, confirmed by an established relationship between brain imaging results and impairment in neurological testing

Appendix B: The Seven Stages of Dementia[79]

I. No impairment of normal function: No signs of memory loss are visible to a medical professional, nor does the patient experience any symptoms.

II. Very mild cognitive decline: People may experience some loss of memory, such as forgetting familiar words, names, or location of wristwatch, eyeglasses, or any such objects of daily use. Family, friends, or colleagues may observe these signs.

III. Mild cognitive decline: Early-stage dementia can be diagnosed only in some individuals with the following symptoms:

- The patient has trouble remembering words or names.
- The patient loses the ability to remember names of individuals newly introduced to him or her.

- Difference in performance can be easily noticeable in work environment, social environment by family, friends, or colleagues.
- Less retention from articles or stories read in a magazine or book.
- The patient misplaces or loses valuable objects.
- Decreased ability to plan or organize.

IV. **Moderate cognitive decline**: Mild or early-stage dementia with the following clear cut deficiencies being observed:

- The patient fails to recollect recent incidents or current events.
- The patient cannot perform some challenging mental arithmetic, such as counting backwards from, say, 100 by 7s.
- The patient is not able to plan or organize complex tasks such as arranging a party or planning a picnic.
- The patient would remain socially withdrawn and silent in challenging situations.

V. **Moderately severe cognitive decline**: It is a moderate or mid-stage AD with major gaps in memory and deficits in cognitive function. Assistance with daily activities may be required and following deficiencies are observed:

- The patient fails to recall current address, telephone number, and name of the college or school from which they graduated.
- The patient is in a confused state of mind with regards to their current location, date, day of the week, season, etc.
- The patient fails to perform even lesser challenging mental arithmetic, such as counting backwards from 40 by 4s.
- The patient requires help in choosing the appropriate clothing for a particular season or occasion.
- Generally, the patient retains substantial knowledge and can tell his or her own name, names of their spouse or children.
- The patients do not require any assistance for eating or using toilet.

VI. Severe cognitive decline: Moderately severe or mid-stage of dementia with memory difficulties continuing to worsen, personality changes emerging substantially and the patients requiring a considerable amount of help for carrying out their day-to-day activities. The following symptoms are observed in the patients:

- The patient loses track of some of the most recent experiences, events, and even their surroundings. The patient cannot recall personal history exactly, though she/he can recall her or his name perfectly. The patient can distinguish familiar faces from unfamiliar faces.

- The patient requires help to dress appropriately, since they tend to create errors such as wearing shoes on the wrong feet.

- The patient experiences a disturbance in normal sleep/ waking cycle.

- The patient would require help for handling the details of toileting such as flushing toilet, wiping, and proper disposal of tissue paper.

- There are increasing episodes of urinary or fecal incontinence.

- Changes in behavior including suspicion and delusions, such as suspecting the care giver as an impostor, hallucinations, repetitive behavior such as hand wringing.

- The patient tends to wander and become lost.

VII. Very severe cognitive decline: Severe or late-stage with the patient losing the ability to respond to the environment, unable to communicate orally, and unable to control movements.

- Very often patients in this stage lose the ability to communicate in a recognizable speech, though they utter phrases occasionally.

- Patients need assistance in eating and toileting, with general incontinence of urine.

- Patients gradually lose the ability to walk without support, to sit, to smile, and hold their head up. Muscles become rigid and reflexes abnormal, with swallowing becoming impaired.

Resources

- Preparing for approaching death: http://www. hospicenet.org/html/preparing_for.html

- Saying goodbye: http://www.hospicenet.org/html/ goodbye-pr.html

- Shake, Rattle, & Roll blog: http://katekelsall.typepad. com/

- Shaky Paws Grampa blog: shakypawsgrampa.blogspot. com

- Mild cognitive impairment: http://www.ncbi.nlm.nih. gov/pmc/articles/PMC2822633/

- Neuropsychological and clinical heterogeneity of cognitive impairment and dementia in patients with Parkinson's disease: http://www.ccs. fau.edu/~bressler/EDU/AdvCogNeuro/pdf/ CogImpairmentParkinson.pdf

- Oxidative stress and neurodegenerative disease: http:// www.ccs.fau.edu/~bressler/EDU/AdvCogNeuro/pdf/ CogImpairmentParkinson.pdf

- Death with Dignity website: http://www. deathwithdignity.org/

- Locate a Movement Disorder Specialist: http://www.pdf.org/en/yy_doctor

- Michael J. Fox Foundation: http://www.michaeljfox.org/

- Parkinson's Disease Foundation: http://www.pdf.org

- National Parkinson Foundation: http://www.parkinson.org/

- Muhammad Ali Parkinson Center Movement Disorder Clinic: http://www.thebarrow.org/Neurological_Services/Muhammad_Ali_Parkinson_Center/index.htm

- American Parkinson's Disease Association: http://www.apdaparkinson.org/userND/%20index.asp

- National Young Onset Center: http://www.youngparkinsons.org/

- Deep brain stimulation information: http://www.medtronic.com/health-consumers/index.htm or http://www.dbs4pd.org/

- International Essential Tremor Foundation: http://www.essentialtremor.org/

- Davis Phinney Foundation: http://www.davisphinneyfoundation.org/

- Parkinson Association of the Rockies: http://www.parkinsonrockies.org/

- Parkinson's organizations and support groups in your area: http://www.pdf.org/en/support_list
- List of Parkinson's organizations worldwide: http://www.pdcaregiver.org/Parkinsons_Organizations.html

Recommended Reading

Alexander, Eban. *Proof of Heaven:* Simon & Schuster, 2012.

Byock, Ira. *Dying Well:* Riverhead Books, 2007.

Dyer, Wayne. *Wisdom of the Ages:* HarperCollins, 1998.

Fox, Michael J. *Lucky Man: A Memoir:* Hyperion, 2002.

Fox, Michael J. *Always Looking Up:* Hyperion, 2009.

Graboys, Thomas. *Life in the Balance:* Union Square, 2008.

Hall, Kirk W. *Carson and His Shaky Paws Grampa:* Innovo Press, 2011.

Hall, Kirk W. *Carina and Her Care Partner Gramma*: Innovo Press, 2013

Hawking, Stephen. *A Brief History of Time*: Bantam, 1998.

Havemann, Joel. *A Life Shaken:* Johns Hopkins, 2002.

Lieberman, Abraham. *Shaking Up Parkinson's Disease: Fighting Like a Tiger, Thinking Like a Fox:* Jones & Bartlett, 2002.

Perlmutter, David. *Grain Brain*: Little, Brown, and Co., 2013.

Whitworth, Helen Buell. *A Caregiver's Guide to Lewy Body Dementia:* Demos Medical Publishing, 2011.

Young, William P. *The Shack:* Windblown Media, 2007.

About the Author

Kirk Hall is a husband, father, and grandfather of six who lives in the Denver area. He has been an author and patient-perspective Parkinson's advocate since 2011. His personal experience as a PWP includes participation in three area support groups, clinical research studies including two visits to the National Institute of Health's National Institute of Neurological Disease & Stroke (NINDS), and joint presentations with movement disorder specialists to support groups sponsored by the Parkinson Association of the Rockies (PAR) and University of Colorado Hospital. Kirk has been a guest speaker at the Muhammad Ali Parkinson Center in Phoenix and has been the subject of television, radio, and newspaper interviews.

He has an undergraduate BS in business from Ohio State and an MBA in Human Resource Development from SUNY at Buffalo. He and his wife of 43 years, Linda, are Parkinson Disease Foundation Clinical Research Advocates. Kirk's *Shaky*

Paws Grampa blog, which includes articles about his writing, advocacy activities, PD-related subjects, and personal journey, can be found at http://shakypawsgrampa.blogspot.com/.

Endnotes

(Endnotes)

1. http://archneur.jamanetwork.com/article.aspx?articleid=791356

2. http://www.alz.org/

3. http://www.ncbi.nlm.nih.gov/pmc/articles/PMC2822633/

4. http://www.dementiaguide.com/aboutdementia/typesofdementia/parkinsons/

5. http://www.nytimes.com/2008/08/26/health/26books.html?_r=0

6. http://www.namenda.com/

7. http://www.exelonpatch.com/index.jsp

8. http://www.ncbi.nlm.nih.gov/pubmed/1736359

9. http://www.pdcaregiver.org/MovementDisorder.html

10. http://www.essentialtremor.org/

11. http://www.spdfoundation.net/about-sensory-processing-disorder.html

12. http://www.dementiaguide.com/aboutdementia/ alzheimers/cognitivereserve/

13. http://www.worldpdcongress.org/

14. http://parkinsons.about.com/od/livingwithpd/a/driving_ with_PD.htm

15. http://www.davisphinneyfoundation.org/living-pd/dvd/

16. http://www.myyogaonline.com/about-yoga/learn-about-yoga/yoga-for-parkinsons-disease

17. http://www.medicalnewstoday.com/articles/250512.php

18. http://www.mindbodygreen.com/0-10979/what-i-wish-everyone-knew-about-parkinsons-disease.html

19. http://uch14.reachlocal.net/conditions/brain-nerves/

20. http://www.thebarrow.org/index.htm

21. http://www.sinemet.org/

22. http://en.wikipedia.org/wiki/Unified_Parkinson's_Disease_ Rating_Scale

23. http://biology.about.com/od/anatomy/p/thalamus.htm

24. http://brain.oxfordjournals.org/content/127/1/4.full.pdf

25. http://www.ninds.nih.gov/

26. http://www.dbssupportgroup.org/history

27. http://en.wikipedia.org/wiki/Neurostimulator

28. http://www.medtronic.com/patients/parkinsons-disease/therapy/index.htm

29. http://en.wikipedia.org/wiki/Montreal_Cognitive_Assessment

30. http://www.michaeljfox.org/understanding-parkinsons/living-with-pd/topic.php%3Falpha-synuclein+&cd=2&hl=en&ct=clnk&gl=us

31. http://en.wikipedia.org/wiki/Lewy_body

32. http://www.parkinson.org/Parkinson-s-Disease/Young-Onset-Parkinsons

33. http://parkinsons.about.com/od/glossary/g/bradyphrenia.htm

34. http://www.dementiaguide.com/aboutdementia/typesofdementia/parkinsons/

35. http://www.lbda.org/node/7

36. http://www.lbda.org/node/470

37. http://www.alz.org/dementia/dementia-with-lewy-bodies-symptoms.asp

38. http://www.medterms.com/script/main/art.asp?articlekey=40362

39. http://www.ncld.org/types-learning-disabilities/executive-function-disorders/what-is-executive- function

40. http://www.britannica.com/EBchecked/topic/374487/memory#toc275815

41. http://www.ccs.fau.edu/~bressler/EDU/AdvCogNeuro/pdf/CogImpairmentParkinson.pdf

42. http://www.mayoclinic.com/health/mild-cognitive-impairment/DS00553

43. http://en.wikipedia.org/wiki/Neuropsychological_assessment

44. https://www.michaeljfox.org/foundation/news-detail.php?michael-fox-foundation-sanofi-launch-clinical-trial-for-drug-to-treat-parkinson-related-cognitive

45. http://www.med.upenn.edu/cndr/donatingbrain.shtml

46. http://www.brightfocus.org/alzheimers/about/understanding/facts.html

47. http://bbrfoundation.org/obama

48. http://www.scientificamerican.com/article.cfm?id=neurostress-how-stress-ma

49. http://www.news-medical.net/health/What-is-Oxidative-Stress.aspx

50. http://www.zonediet.com/blog/2012/01/what-is-cellular-inflammation/

51. https://docs.google.com/gview?url=http://cdn.intechopen.com/pdfs/24872.pdf&embedded=true&time=0444557309ab06b99a399b3fe6b78c5f

52. http://www.webmd.com/food-recipes/features/how-antioxidants-work1

53. http://www.nia.nih.gov/alzheimers/publication/alzheimers-disease-genetics-fact-sheet

54. http://www.simplypsychology.org/maslow.html

55. http://professionaldestiny.com/2009/10/08/career-dissonance/

56. http://psychology.about.com/od/psychologicaltesting/a/myers-briggs-type-indicator.htm

57. http://www.typelogic.com/infj.html

58. http://thoreau.eserver.org/walden00.html

59. http://www.lbda.org/content/diagnosis

60. http://www.alz.org/dementia/dementia-with-lewy-bodies-symptoms.asp

61. http://www.johnshopkinshealthalerts.com/alerts/memory/Benefits-of-Staying-Mentally-Active_6343-1.html

62. http://www.youtube.com/watch?v=Y10VEkyKd3w

63. http://www.ncbi.nlm.nih.gov/pubmed/18582232

64. http://en.wikipedia.org/wiki/Strategic_planning

65. http://en.wikipedia.org/wiki/Management_by_objectives

66. http://sbinfocanada.about.com/od/marketing/g/targetmarketing.htm

67. http://searchcio.techtarget.com/definition/Total-Quality-Management

68. http://searchcrm.techtarget.com/definition/CRM

69. http://www.businessdictionary.com/definition/customer-centric.html

70. http://www.balancedpolitics.org/universal_health_care.htm

71. http://money.usnews.com/money/blogs/the-best-life/2011/02/25/how-to-ensure-your-last-wishes-are-carried-out

72. http://www.enchantedlearning.com/subjects/astronomy/stars/lifecycle/

73. http://curious.astro.cornell.edu/stars.php

74. http://www.enchantedlearning.com/subjects/astronomy/stars/lifecycle/stardeath.shtml

75. http://www.world-science.net/othernews/121102_EBL.htm

76. http://www.dementiaguide.com/aboutdementia/typesofdementia/parkinsons/

77. http://www.lbda.org/node/7

78. http://www.lbda.org/node/470

79. http://livingwithlewybodyebook.blogspot.com/2008/03/
stages-of-lbd-and-lewy-update.html